Minor Trauma in Child...

A po...

Ffion C W Davies MRCPCH, FFAEM
A&E Consultant, The Royal London Hospital

with contributions from

W Joan Robson FRCS, FFAEM

and

Alison K Smith MRCP, FFAEM

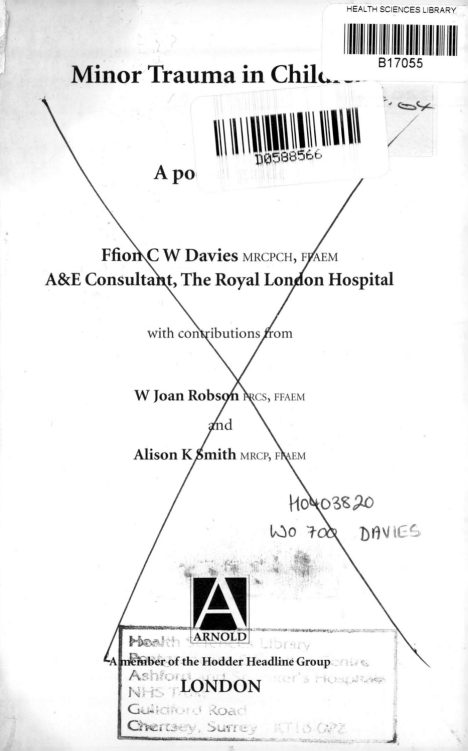

ARNOLD

A member of the Hodder Headline Group

LONDON

First published in Great Britain in 2003 by
Arnold, a member of the Hodder Headline Group,
338 Euston Road, London NW1 3BH

http://www.arnoldpublishers.com

Distributed in the United States of America by
Oxford University Press Inc.,
198 Madison Avenue, New York, NY10016
Oxford is a registered trademark of Oxford University Press

British Library Cataloguing in Publication Data
A catalogue record for this book is available from the British Library

Library of Congress Cataloging-in-Publication Data
A catalog record for this book is available from the Library of Congress

ISBN   0 340 73204 0

1 2 3 4 5 6 7 8 9 10

Commissioning Editor:	Joanna Koster
Development Editor:	Sarah Burrows
Project Editor:	James Rabson
Production Controller:	Deborah Smith
Cover Design:	Terry Griffiths

Typeset in Minion by Phoenix Photosetting, Chatham, Kent
Printed and bound in Malta

What do you think about this book? Or any other Arnold title? Please send your
comments to feedback.arnold@hodder.co.uk

Contents

Preface

As the sub-speciality of paediatric emergency medicine grows, so does the literature to support it. There is now plenty of help out there for health professionals to learn about medical emergencies or major trauma in children. But information about the little things in life can be the hardest to find – the things that cause the majority of parents to take their child to an emergency department at some time.

This book is meant as an easy reference book for busy doctors and nurses, in hospitals, minor injury units or family practice. It contains information in an easy to find, easy to read format. It covers everything from foreign bodies up the nose to orthopaedics. The authors have drawn upon their own experience and included helpful hints gleaned over years of practice, which are rarely written down formally in books.

 Stop signs within the text indicate where the subject is beyond the scope of the book and may be beyond the reader's experience.

 Warning signs indicate potential pitfalls.

F Davies
January 2003

Acknowledgements

I would like to thank the following people: Tim Coats for his endless patience and advice, Bill Coode for solving my imaging nightmares, and all the children who were so willing to act as models for the photographs – Darnell McPherson, Derisha McPherson, Scott Linney, Nathan Smith, Carley Smith and Madeline Coode.

1

Introduction

Children comprise between 20–35% of all patients attending a general emergency department (ED). In the UK it is also estimated that in any one year around 2.3 million children visit the ED as a result of injury: this translates to around a fifth of all children. The impact, therefore, of children on emergency services and, likewise, the impact of emergency services on children, is enormous. Children are likely to have repeated attendances at an ED, and the care that they receive influences both the initial presentation and future attendances.

The purpose of this book is to enable doctors, nurses and emergency nurse practitioners to manage common minor injuries, to know when to ask for help, and to spot when the minor injury is only the tip of the iceberg, so to speak. It is relevant for practitioners based in hospitals, minor injury units and primary care centres. Similarly, although aimed at a UK audience, much of it will be relevant to other countries. It is not an exhaustive text and, in this evidence-based world in which we now live, much is written on the basis of experience. Minor injuries are one of the poorest-researched areas of medicine and the quality of the scientific literature is generally poor.

A child's minor injury should not be seen in isolation. The whole spectrum of the child's development, family and life experience is important, and the episode should be managed in a manner that is efficient, pleasurable and educative. Although the professional might define an injury as 'minor', the effects on the child and family may be considerable, not least a visit to an ED itself! Children should be seen in an area audiovisually separated from adults. This area should be specifically designed for their needs with child-sized equipment, suitable play areas, and examination and treatment rooms that are bright and welcoming and reflect children's own familiar environment. It is quite easy to transform an area with brightly coloured paint and posters, and funding is often readily available from local charities.

A well-designed department can also help with the assessment and treatment of children: in particular, the use of a play area, visible from the main working area. The importance of play in the assessment and treatment of children should be taught to all staff. Toys can be used as distraction therapy during painful procedures, as tools for examination, and as entertainment during observation or waiting times. Maintaining a stock of playthings is often difficult, as they inevitably seem to disappear from a department, and a constant supply is necessary. Staff should be encouraged to bring in their own children's outgrown toys, and local businesses may be happy to provide donations. Larger departments may employ a play therapist. This person can identify suitable play tools, ameliorate the atmosphere of the waiting area, and usefully prepare children for procedures and the hospital environment.

Children are usually accompanied by parents, siblings and/or a variety of assorted company. A family waiting room needs to be far larger than may be thought necessary for the numbers of patients seen! Facilities to assuage boredom, such as a television and/or video and vending machines, are also useful. The area may need to be used for the children of ill or injured parents.

All ED doctors and nurses have experience of dealing with children's problems. It is recommended that departments that see more than 18 000 children per year have both a lead consultant and 24-hour nursing cover, all of whom have additional training in paediatrics. There needs to be close liaison between emergency medicine staff and paediatricians, and it is recommended that a consultant paediatrician acts as a designated link for advice, teaching and development of guidelines. Clinicians with a paediatric background will need to develop the emergency aspect of their specialty. Emergency specialists can offer expertise in trauma and adolescent issues.

The word 'children' does not define a homogenous group. The facilities and skills needed to deal with babies are very different to those required for adolescents. A wide range of sizes and type of equipment are needed. It is important that staff are aware of the particular size of kit needed, and charts of ET tube sizes and drug dosages are essential.

Emergency departments need to have a strong awareness and proper protocols for dealing with non-accidental injury, as it is often here that suspicions are first raised about a child's well-being. They may also have other functions as well as the reception, assessment and treatment of acutely ill or injured children. Many run review clinics for the child's injury to be reassessed or redressed. These clinic areas must also be child friendly and it is often here where the benefits of a comfortable first visit are recognized. EDs can provide a vital role in the prevention of children being admitted to hospital with the use of observation beds (e.g. for accidental overdose, minor head injury, etc.) or outreach nurses, who follow up children with a home visit.

Prevention of injury

INTRODUCTION

'Accidents' are the commonest cause of death in children aged 1–15 years in the UK. Injury is also a leading cause of ill health and disability in this age group, causing around 10 000 children to become permanently disabled every year. Many injuries in children presenting to the emergency department (ED) could have been avoided by adequate supervision and common sense measures, so in a sense are not truly 'accidents'. There is a marked association between age and location of the injury. Healthy living for children must include physical activities and the gradual development of independence; therefore, injuries are inevitable during this period. To minimize the incidence and the severity of injuries, children and young people must be in environments that are safe, while giving fun and freedom.

Most injuries to children less than 3 years of age occur in the home or garden. At this age, children develop rapidly and carers often underestimate their capabilities. Although it is impossible to have 'eyes in the back of your head' when looking after small children, it is important that true neglect is not missed (see Chapter 15 'Non-accidental Injury'). When children become older, they attend nurseries or schools, and move further from home for play and other activities. Many incidents leading to injury then occur in schools, sports facilities, in official playgrounds or in derelict buildings, on roads, farms and at work.

There is also a strong association between injury rates and social class. For example, children in social class 5 are seven times more likely to die in a pedestrian road accident than those in social class 1.

All parents, carers, children and young people, and health care professionals should use every opportunity to be active in injury prevention programmes in the classical areas of: education, engineering and enforcement (legislation).

EDUCATION

The role of teachers

Injury awareness and first aid skills can be incorporated into most parts of the school curriculum and information to support these sessions can come from local EDs, the emergency services and rail service personnel. This can be complemented by visits to EDs. A successful example of this approach is the Injury Minimization Project for Schools (IMPS), which is aimed at year 6 children.

Parents, carers and children themselves

Most research on injury prevention indicates that it is difficult to bring about behavioural changes; however, motivation is high in the context of acute injury. Health care professionals should take advantage of this to try to prevent recurrence of the incident that led to the injury. Parents are more receptive to advice about cycle helmets when their child has just fallen off a bike, or to the suggestion that drugs should be locked away in a drug cupboard after an accidental overdose. Leaflets on these subjects can be made available in the ED, and educational videos can be played in the waiting areas.
  Key subjects are:
- safety equipment, e.g. stair gates and fireguards;
- child-resistant containers for medicines;
- safe storage of household cleaners and garden products;
- safe positioning of hot objects, e.g. cups of tea, kettles, pans and irons;
- safe use of equipment, e.g. not to put baby bouncers on work surfaces, and always supervise the use of babywalkers;
- safety on roads and railways.

The role of health visitors

Health visitors have a key role in injury prevention. At routine assessments and in clinic visits, they can give out information leaflets and discuss the development of the child in relation to injury prevention. On home visits, they can give constructive advice on hazards in the home. National guidance recommends that health visitors should receive notification of all ED attendances in small children.

ENGINEERING

Knowledge of child development and the potential for injury should be included in the training of all designers, architects and engineers. The design of every home, public building, playground and highway, and manufacturers of all consumer products should take into account the fact that children may be injured by their products. If a doctor or nurse becomes aware of a hazard that has led to the injury of a child, this should be discussed with a senior doctor. With parental permission, this can then be reported to the appropriate agency, e.g. the local authority, Trading Standards Office, Health and Safety Executive or Member of Parliament, for action.

ENFORCEMENT (LEGISLATION)

To be effective, legislation must be realistic and enforceable. Examples that have been beneficial in reducing injury are the legislation on child-resistant containers, and on the wearing of seatbelts and the restraint of children in cars.

Audit and research in emergency departments can support or denounce the need for new legislation or a change in legislation. Health care professionals are in a good position to suggest subjects for audit and research based on the patterns of injury they see in their clinical work. The seat belt laws and European Standards on consumer products are good examples of changes that have been supported by accurate information from EDs.

Pain management

INTRODUCTION

The vast majority of minor injuries cause some degree of pain. Recognition and alleviation of pain should be a priority when treating injuries. This process should ideally start at the triage point and finish with ensuring that adequate analgesia is provided at discharge.

On the whole, pain is commonly under-recognized and undertreated in children. There are several reasons for this. In particular, assessing pain in children can be difficult. Children in pain may be quiet and withdrawn, rather than crying. Also there is often insecurity about dosage of medication in children. There is a myth that children feel less pain than adults but this is not true: even neonates and fetuses feel pain.

Communication may be difficult with an upset child, and it may be difficult to distinguish pain from other causes of distress (e.g. fear, stranger anxiety, etc.). Some words are better understood than others, depending on what words the family use, e.g. hurt, sore, poorly. In some cases, children may deny pain for fear of the ensuing treatment (particularly needles).

ASSESSMENT OF PAIN

(STOP) **Think ... if pain is severe, is it major injury or ischaemia?**

Your prior experience of injuries can help in estimating the amount of pain the child is likely to be in. For example, a fractured shaft of femur or a burn are more painful than a bump on the head. Beyond that, in young (non-verbal) children, we can only rely on visual clues, such as crying or loss of movement of a limb, which can be measured by behavioural scoring systems, such as the CHEOPS score.

Pain assessment now forms an integral part of the National Triage Guidelines. The pain ladder used in the guidelines uses descriptive and numerical scales. The Advanced Paediatric Life Support (APLS) course pain ladder (Advanced Life Support Group Ltd) incorporates panda faces, and some scales are based solely on faces, such as the Wong Baker faces.

However, children may have difficulty in applying abstract concepts, such as numbers or pictures, to their pain, or may have reasons for either downplaying or exaggerating their pain, so we suggest a composite score rather than relying on one system. Figure 3.1 shows a suggested pain assessment tool, which is currently being validated for use in the ED. The assessor uses the available information to decide on the category of the pain.

WHAT ARE WE TREATING?

- *Pain* This requires analgesia (see below).
- *Fear* All efforts should be made to provide a calm, friendly environment. You should explain what you are doing, preparing the child for any procedures, and let the parents stay with the child unless they prefer not to or are particularly distressed.
- *Loss of control* Children like to be involved in decisions and feel that they are being listened to.
- *Focus on injury* Distraction and other cognitive techniques are extremely useful (see below).

HOW TO TREAT PAIN

Having assessed the degree of pain, there is a range of ways to treat it. This includes psychological strategies, non-pharmacological adjuncts and pharmacological agents, via various routes. A working knowledge of all the options is useful, so that your treatment is appropriate for the child's age, injury and degree of pain. A suggested strategy for common conditions is given in Table 3.1.

	No pain	Mild pain	Moderate pain	Severe pain
Faces scale score (circle)	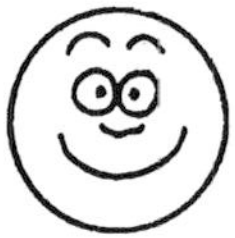	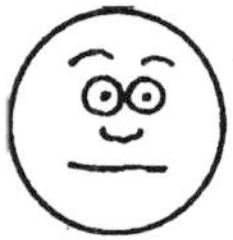	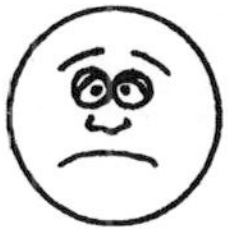	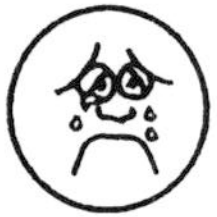
Number score (circle)	0	1–4	5–7	8–10
Behaviour (circle each relevant observation)	Normal activity No ↓ movement Happy	Rubbing affected area Decreased movement Neutral expression Able to play/talk normally	Protective of affected area ↓ movement/quiet Complaining of pain Consolable crying Grimaces when affected part moved/touched	No movement or defensive of affected part Looking frightened Very quiet Restless, unsettled Complaining of lots of pain Inconsolable crying
Injury example	Bump on head	Abrasion Small laceration Sprain ankle/knee # fingers/clavical Sore throat	Small burn/scald Fingertip injury # forearm/elbow/ankle	Large burn # long bone/dislocation Appendicitis Sickle crisis
Category chosen (tick)				

Figure 3.1 Pain assessment too .

Table 3.1 Examples of strategies for managing pain in common injuries (see also Chapter 17 'Practical Procedures').

Injury	Psychological strategies	Non-pharmacological adjuncts	Pharmacological strategies
Facial wound	√	Consider conscious sedation.	Oral paracetamol. Local anaesthesia.
Fractured femur	√	Sling, splint or plaster backslab	Entonox as interim measure. Intranasal diamorphine or intravenous morphine. Femoral or '3 in 1' nerve block.
Burn	√	Initial cooling, then cover with dressing or cling wrap	Minor – oral paracetamol and / or ibuprofen Major – intranasal diamorphine or intravenous morphine
Minor head injury	√	Cold compress	Oral paracetamol and/or ibuprofen

Psychological strategies

Psychological strategies should be relevant to the age of child, but are useful in all situations. Experienced staff are invaluable when handling distressed children. It is important to be reassuring but sympathetic. Cuddling, stroking and talking to children helps to reassure them. Simply explaining what you are going to do will help the child gain confidence in you.

Distraction can be provided by toys, blowing bubbles, murals on walls, reading or story-telling using superhero or magical imagery to make the pain go away. Hypnosis is successful but is a skill that has to be learned. Music is both soothing and distracting. Videos are useful, although turning one off before it has finished can be tricky!

Non-pharmacological adjuncts

Splintage of injured limbs, and elevation of the lower leg above hip level or elevation of the hand in a high arm sling (see Chapter 17 'Practical Procedures' reduce swelling and, therefore, pain. When treating burns, reducing air currents with cling wrap or dressings is sometimes all that is needed. Regular application of ice packs (e.g. frozen peas) to soft tissue injuries reduces inflammation (avoiding direct contact of ice with skin). Small children dislike ice packs but a bowl of cool water can be tried.

Pharmacological agents

 For major injuries, seek senior advice and obtain IV access.

Figure 3.2 demonstrates a suggested algorithm for the treatment of mild, moderate and severe pain.

Oral medication
- *Mild pain* may be treated with paracetamol or non-steroidal anti-inflammatory drugs, such as ibuprofen. A combination of both is often successful.
- *Moderate pain* may be treated with codeine-containing preparations.
- *More severe pain* may be treated with oral morphine solution (Oramorph™) but this takes around 20 minutes to start working. A useful alternative with a quicker onset of action is intranasal diamorphine (see below).

Intranasal analgesia
Intranasal diamorphine has a rapid onset of action (2–5 minutes) and is highly effective. Its use is becoming popular for the following reasons: it acts much quicker than oral opiates, is well tolerated, avoids a needle and has marked anxiolytic effects. Its offset is around 30 minutes, by which time dressings or splints will have been applied and the child's trust gained, so that, if ongoing analgesia is needed, insertion of an intravenous (IV) line is much easier and less traumatic (see the chart in Table 3.2 for full dosage and administration). 0.1 mg/kg is made up to 0.2 ml with water and dropped into the nostril using a 1 ml syringe with the head tilted back slightly.

Inhalational analgesia
Nitrous oxide and oxygen (Entonox™) can be provided in cylinders with a facemask or intraoral delivery system. It depends on the child's cooperation and coordination, and understanding that it is self-activated. For continuous administration, see 'Conscious sedation' (below).

 Nitrous oxide should not be used for children with head injuries or injuries to the chest with a risk of pneumothorax.

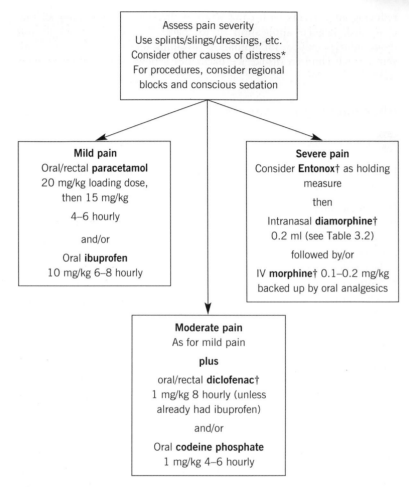

Assess pain severity
Use splints/slings/dressings, etc.
Consider other causes of distress*
For procedures, consider regional
blocks and conscious sedation

Mild pain
Oral/rectal **paracetamol**
20 mg/kg loading dose,
then 15 mg/kg
4–6 hourly

and/or

Oral **ibuprofen**
10 mg/kg 6–8 hourly

Severe pain
Consider **Entonox**† as holding
measure

then

Intranasal **diamorphine**†
0.2 ml (see Table 3.2)

followed by/or

IV **morphine**† 0.1–0.2 mg/kg
backed up by oral analgesics

Moderate pain
As for mild pain

plus

oral/rectal **diclofenac**†
1 mg/kg 8 hourly (unless
already had ibuprofen)

and/or

Oral **codeine phosphate**
1 mg/kg 4–6 hourly

*Other causes of distress include: fear of the unfamiliar environment, parental distress, stranger anxiety, needle phobia, fear of injury severity.
†**Contraindications:**
Ibuprofen/diclofenac: avoid if previous reactions to NSAIDs or in moderate or severe asthmatics.
Entonox: avoid in head injury, or chest injury with risk of pneumothorax.
Intravenous morphine: use with caution if risk of depression of airway, breathing or circulation.

Figure 3.2 Algorithm for the treatment of pain (based on pain score).

Table 3.2 Dosage of intranasal diamorphine for acute pain. Dilute 10 mg of diamorphine powder with the specific volume of water. Instil 0.2 ml of the solution into one nostril, using a 1 ml syringe (gives 0.1 mg/kg in 0.2 ml).

Child's weight (kg)	Volume of water (ml)
10	1.9
15	1.3
20	1.0
25	0.8
30	0.7
35	0.6
40	0.5
50	0.4
60	0.3

Topical anaesthesia

Lignocaine gel is useful for dirty abrasions that need to be cleaned. Local anaesthetic creams such as Ametop™ or EMLA™ are not licensed for use on open wounds, and have an onset of action of 30–60 minutes, so are of limited use for other urgent situations. However, if time allows, it is useful to use these before local infiltration of anaesthesia.

Local infiltration of anaesthesia

Infiltration of local anaesthetic is painful and may not be justified if only one or two sutures are required. The pain is reduced by using a narrow bore needle (e.g. dental needle) and by slow injection (see Chapter 17 'Practical Procedures').

Regional anaesthesia

Nerve blocks are easy to learn, well tolerated by children, and avoid the risks of sedation and respiratory depression. Particularly useful nerve blocks are the femoral or 'three-in-one' nerve blocks for a fractured femur, the infra-auricular block for removing earrings and digital nerve blocks for fingers (see Chapter 17 'Practical Procedures').

Intravenous analgesia

Intravenous opiates such as morphine are used when immediate analgesia is required. There should be no hesitation in administering these drugs to children provided care is taken and resuscitation facilities are available.

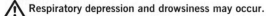 **Respiratory depression and drowsiness may occur.**

This may be avoided by titrating from a small dose to an adequate dose over a few minutes. Naloxone should be available for reversal, if necessary. Antiemetics are not usually required in young children.

Intramuscular (IM) route

This route is best avoided as it subjects the child to a needle and holds no advantage over the IV route. Absorption is unpredictable and often slow, making repeated doses (and, therefore, needles) necessary and the dosage difficult to calculate.

CONSCIOUS SEDATION/ANXIOLYSIS

In order to perform some procedures, an anxiolytic agent is useful. A wider discussion of the various techniques for conscious sedation is beyond the scope of this handbook. Conscious sedation holds benefits for the child (amnesia and avoidance of generating fear for subsequent hospital treatment), the child's parents, other parents and children who might otherwise hear screams, the staff and, importantly, a more thorough and better technical result for the procedure itself.

(STOP) **Adequate monitoring, trained staff and resuscitation facilities are essential. Do not attempt conscious sedation unless your unit fulfils the basic require ments and your consultant approves its use.**

The American College of Emergency Physicians Guidelines recommend one-to-one nursing, a doctor experienced in paediatric airway management, monitoring and resuscitation equipment (see 'Further reading').

Midazolam is a benzodiazepine, which may be given orally, intranasally, rectally or intravenously. Oral midazolam at a dose of 0.5 mg/kg provides mild anxiolysis within 10–15 minutes, but has wide individual variation in effect and can cause hyperactivity. It is most useful in facilitating distraction, such as when removing a foreign body. The oral route is less likely to cause a rapid peak in drug levels than the rectal route, and is better tolerated than the intranasal route, which may cause local irritation. *N.B. It is not an analgesic.*

Nitrous oxide 50% , with 50% oxygen administered continuously provides analgesia, anxiolysis and amnesia. Monitoring and resuscitation facilities are needed.

Ketamine is a useful alternative that provides 'dissociative anaesthesia'. This has a good safety profile and may be given IV or IM. Upper respiratory tract symptoms or abnormal airway anatomy (e.g. history of prolonged ventilation) are a contraindication to the use of ketamine. A dose of 4 mg/kg IM, or 1–2 mg/kg IV, works within 5 minutes and allows you to perform procedures lasting up to 30 minutes with the child remaining very still and undistressed. The IV route allows you to titrate the dose and wears off quicker.

Ketamine may cause hypersalivation, which, rarely, may cause laryngospasm. A total of 0.02 mg/kg atropine should, therefore, be given in addition. Also, children over 10 years old are at risk of agitation and hallucinations in the 'emergence' phase as the drug wears off. Older children should, therefore, be allowed to recover in a quiet room.

Further reading

1. Advanced Life Support Group: *Management of pain in children. Advanced paediatric life support manual*, 3rd edn. London: BMJ Books, 2001.
2. American College of Emergency Physicians Policy Statement: The use of pediatric sedation and analgesia. *Ann Emerg Med* 1993;22:626–627.
3. *Emergency triage*. London: BMJ Publishing Group, 1997.
4. Krauss B: Management of acute pain and anxiety in children undergoing procedures in the emergency department. *Ped Emerg Care* 2001;17:115–122.

Wounds and soft tissue injuries

INTRODUCTION

Wounds and superficial injuries form a large part of paediatric trauma. Wounds, in particular, are a source of anxiety for children, parents and emergency department staff. Often the child is distressed by the accident itself, the parents are concerned about scarring, and both parents and staff may be reticent about the procedure of wound repair itself.

Many of these difficulties can be overcome if you understand the mechanism of injury (take a good history), the nature of the wound (knowledge of anatomy and wound healing) and the options for satisfactory repair. The use of psychological techniques, a well-trained nurse and adequate analgesia will make the procedure more endurable for all (see Chapter 3 'Pain Management').

BASIC HISTORY

Important questions

Mechanism

A detailed history is needed to alert you to potential problems.

 The injury may be part of a greater picture that may herald more major injuries.

For example:
- underlying injury to bones, tendons or nerves;
- significant head injury;
- significant blood loss;
- deliberate self-harm;
- non-accidental injury.

Time of injury

Wounds over 12 hours old may be better left to heal by secondary intention. If the wound is clean and neat, it may be repaired for up to 24 hours, particularly if it is on the face or scalp.

Tetanus immunization status

Most children in the UK currently will be covered for tetanus. Children in the UK are routinely immunized at 2,3 and 4 months old, then again pre-school and aged 14–15. Each booster, from the pre-school vaccination, provides 10 years of immunity. If that period has been exceeded *and* the wound is dirty, anti-tetanus immunoglobulin may be given. Otherwise, a further booster is advisable. If a child is not immunized, some emergency departments offer opportunistic immunization, but this has to be agreed locally, so that duplication does not occur.

Concurrent illness

This is rarely an issue in children and does not usually affect wound repair, although there may be a history of, for example, immunosuppression or long-term steroid treatment. Also children with chronic illness may be more frightened of needles.

Allergies

Document allergies, particularly to penicillin or tape and dressings.

Consideration of non-accidental injury and accident prevention

The circumstances of the accident need to be given adequate attention (see Chapter 15 'Non-accidental Injury'). However, wounds usually raise concerns more about supervision of the child than actual deliberate injury. The health visitor should be notified for all injuries to pre-school children. They will identify issues around accident prevention and may subsequently visit the family at home.

BASIC EXAMINATION AND WOUND DESCRIPTION

Description of wound

Site

Be aware of the anatomical structures underlying the wound. *Bleeding* can be significant from scalp wounds and those involving arteries and arterioles. *Healing* is quickest in wounds on the face and scalp, and slowest in those on the legs or over joints. It is worth considering splintage for knee and heel wounds, for example. *Infection* is more likely in dirty areas of the body, e.g. soles of the feet. Always *draw diagrams,* which are clearer than text, and measure and describe accurately, for medicolegal purposes.

Size

Large wounds may need suturing under general anaesthesia, as they may require more than the maximum safe dose of local anaesthetic.

Depth

This will affect the likelihood of damage to underlying structures and your options for closure (see below).

Assessment for complications

Deep penetrating wounds

Stab wounds, e.g. from scissors, knives, etc., often penetrate deeper than is obvious. Gunshot wounds inflict severe injury and require expert management.

 Seek senior advice immediately. Treat A, B, C, D, before focusing on the wound.

Neurovascular and motor complications

A knowledge of anatomy is required to assess for potential damage to underlying structures. Assessment is difficult in pre-verbal children.

The skin surrounding and distal to the wound should be normal in colour, have normal sensation, and pulses and capillary refill should be formally tested. Full motor power against resistance should be tested for muscle groups and tendons. Pain and lack of use can cause pallor and sweating acutely, particularly in the hands and feet of teenagers, and is caused by autonomic changes; this is innocent. Any other abnormalities should be referred to a surgeon for assessment.

⚠ If in doubt, always seek expert advice.

FACTORS INVOLVED IN HEALING

Wounds generally heal better in children than adults. However the wound appears in the first month, you should advise that both improvement in the appearance and worsening due to scar contraction are possible. Children with pigmented skins may have hypopigmentation of the affected area, either for a year or so, or long term. Those of Afro-Caribbean origin may develop keloid scars. Many wounds itch when healing and simple moisturizers (particularly those used for treating eczema) are useful. Sun sensitivity may be a problem for 6–12 months, so recommend protective creams.

Site and time of injury

See 'Basic history' and 'Basic examination and wound description' (above).

Skin tension lines

Delayed healing and/or scarring are most likely when wounds are under tension. Langer's lines (see Figures 4.1 and 4.2) describe the lines of natural tension in the body. If a wound is aligned with these lines, healing occurs quicker and is less likely to produce a scar than wounds that cross the lines.

Dirty wounds/infection

Organic material is far more likely to cause infection than inorganic material. Clearly, substances such as soil carry a high bacterial load. Also, bacteria multiply in a logarithmic fashion so the longer a wound remains dirty, the higher the risk.

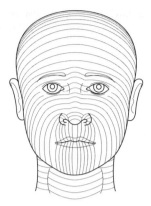

Figure 4.1 Langer's lines of the face.

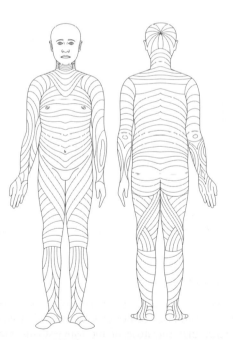

Figure 4.2 Langer's lines of the body.

Crush injury

Crush injuries are more likely to produce swelling and ragged edges, which are difficult to oppose, causing delayed healing and scarring. They may also damage the skin, causing haematoma formation and jeopardizing viability.

Vascularity of wound

Any areas whose blood supply is jeopardized may not heal, or will scar. Dead material also provides a haven for infection. If tissues are clearly dead, they should be debrided. However, skin in children may look non-viable but often survives, so should not be debrided but reviewed after a few days. Seek senior advice.

Foreign bodies (see also Chapter 13 'Foreign Bodies')

Foreign bodies such as grit and oil may cause tattooing if left (see 'Abrasions' below).

⚠ Always consider the potential presence of a foreign body in any infected wound.

⚠ Always request a soft tissue X-ray if an injury has been caused by glass.

Most types of glass are radio-opaque. Fragments are notoriously difficult to spot with the naked eye, and may lie deep. If glass has been removed from a wound, a follow-up X-ray must be performed.

GENERAL MANAGEMENT

Abrasions

Abrasions may be of variable depth, and can be described and treated in a similar way to burns. In children, abrasions may be contaminated with road tar, which has the potential to cause 'tattooing'. If the wound is inadequately cleaned, dirt particles become ingrained and cause permanent disfigurement.

At initial presentation, every attempt must be made to make the wound as clean as possible, using local anaesthesia (gel or infiltrated) if necessary. Forceps, surgical brushes or needles may be used. If the surface area to be cleaned is so large that the dose of local anaesthetic may be exceeded, general anaesthesia may be necessary.

If a little dirt remains, this may work its way out over the next few days, and dressings and creams such as those used to deslough chronic ulcers may be helpful. Follow-up is necessary.

 Do not leave the wound dirty for more than 2 or 3 days. If difficulties persist, refer to a general or plastic surgeon.

Cleaning and irrigation of wounds

The majority of wounds may be considered dirty, but those contaminated with organic material are particularly at risk of infection. Good wound toilet, with adequate dilution of the bacterial load with copious water, is far more important than relying on prophylactic antibiotics (see Chapter 17 'Practical Procedures').

Exploration of wounds

Exploration of a wound should be considered when a foreign body or damage to underlying structures is suspected. However, it should be remembered that children poorly tolerate several injections to create an anaesthetic field, or prolonged periods of wound exploration. Further, this should not be undertaken if it is clear at the outset that more experienced help is needed. Lastly, do not extend a wound without seeking advice first.

WOUND REPAIR
(see also Chapter 17 'Practical Procedures')

See Chapter 17 for details on the application of adhesive strips and glue, anaesthesia, local infiltration and regional blocks, and insertion of sutures.

Primary repair or not?

Wounds over 12 hours old (24 hours for facial or scalp wounds), those which are contaminated, contused, devitalised, or bites, are more likely to become infected, and are best left open, to heal by granulation and eventual re-epithelialisation. In such wounds, sutures act as an additional foreign body and increase the risk of infection; opposition of the wound edges (either by sutures or adhesive strips) makes the underlying wound anaerobic and more prone to infection. You should consider prescribing an antibiotic, such as flucloxacillin, if suturing an injury below the neck after 12 hours.

Wounds with skin loss should also usually be allowed to heal by secondary intention, rather than creating tension by trying to achieve primary closure. Wounds with skin loss of less than a square centimetre tend to do well, and even larger areas will often heal in children, without recourse to skin grafting. In certain circumstances, delayed primary closure after 4–5 days is appropriate – seek surgical advice.

Choice of technique for wound closure

While interrupted sutures are often perceived as the gold standard in wound repair, in fact the cosmetic result is as good with adhesive strips and/or glue, provided there is no tension on the wound. Factors such as Langer's lines (see 'Factors involved in healing' above) are more important than depth. It is important, however, not to avoid sutures if they are indicated, simply because of the practical difficulties of suturing uncooperative children.

AFTERCARE

Dressings

The purpose of a dressing is to prevent additional contamination of the wound, and to provide a barrier to air currents and friction against clothing, etc. Wounds that are oozing (blood or serous fluid) must be dressed with a non-stick dressing, so that changing the dressing in the next day or two does not hurt, or disturb the wound too much. Paraffin-impregnated gauze is a suitable dressing.

After the first 24–72 hours, silicon-based or other non-stick dressings, or even dry dressings can be used. It is best to leave the wound undisturbed for a few days, unless it is at high risk of infection. Unfortunately, despite tape, children often pull dressings off, or get them wet or dirty, necessitating more frequent dressing changes.

A more detailed discussion of wound dressing is too large a topic to be covered in this book, and there is a great deal of variation, depending on local circumstances.

Antibiotics

Good wound toilet (see above) is more important than antibiotic treatment. Antibiotics are only necessary if there is a high risk of infection (see below). An anti-staphylococcal and anti-streptococcal agent such as flucloxacillin is appropriate. Gram-negative cover is only needed for certain animal bites (see Chapter 12 'Bites, Stings and Allergic Reactions'), oral or perineal wounds, or those sustained in muddy areas or water.

Tetanus

See 'Basic history' (above).

Immobilization

If a wound is over a mobile area such as a joint, wound healing is often speeded up considerably, and scarring reduced, if the part is immobilized. Since children are less prone to stiffness than adults, a splint or small plaster of Paris is often useful.

Suture removal

If sutures are left in too long, there is an increased risk of infection and suture marks remaining on the skin long-term. Children heal much quicker than adults, so sutures can usually be removed on day 4 on the face, and day 5 on other areas, unless under tension. The wound can always be supported by adhesive strips for a few days after sutures are removed.

COMMON COMPLICATIONS

Infection

Infection is more likely in wounds that are dirty or contain a foreign body, those with contused or crushed skin, puncture wounds, or those with a delay in treatment or cleaning. It may sometimes be difficult to tell if a wound is infected but signs include slow healing, ongoing oozing, surrounding erythema, smell, fever and pain. Wound swabs do not yield useful microbiological results for 2–3 days so the decision to treat is usually clinical.

If a wound becomes infected, consider the presence of a foreign body. Treat with an antibiotic such as flucloxacillin, immobilize it or discourage use of the limb, elevate it if possible, and remove sutures if present. Spreading cellulitis, lymphangitis or systemic upset are indications for intravenous antibiotics.

⚠ **Infected wounds should be reviewed after a day.**

Dehiscence

If dehiscence occurs, seek surgical advice. Dehiscence is more likely in the presence of wound infection.

SPECIFIC WOUNDS AND AREAS

Puncture wounds

Innocent-looking puncture wounds are a minefield to the unwary. Firstly, they may be much deeper than initially suspected, and a thorough clinical examination of underlying structures should be undertaken (see beginning of chapter). Secondly, bacteria are injected deep into tissues. The smaller the wound, the more likely it is to become infected because the overlying skin edges are opposed. Consider prophylactic antibiotics and review after 24–48 hours.

Needlestick injuries

Hospitals often have their own needlestick policy. Children may sustain such injuries when they find discarded needles in areas inhabited by drug misusers. If you have no local policy, advise parents that the risk of blood-borne infection is low, but is higher for hepatitis B than human immuno-deficiency virus (HIV). Also post-exposure prophylaxis for potential hepatitis B infection carries minimal side-effects, unlike HIV. Seek specialist advice.

Fishhooks

See Chapter 13 'Foreign Bodies'.

Plantar wounds of the foot

These wounds are notorious for their propensity to develop infection, particularly *Pseudomonas aeruginosa*, often after a delay of several days to a few weeks. Patients should be advised to return if foot pain increases, and appropriate specialist advice sought if this occurs.

HAIR TOURNIQUET SYNDROME

History

This odd syndrome occurs when one or more hairs become wrapped around a digit, and gradually constrict, causing ischaemia. It is most common in toddlers and babies. Extremely close examination may be needed to find the hair, but it is usually easily recognized if you are familiar with the condition.

Examination

The digit may be bluish or white. A magnifying glass may be needed to see the hair(s).

Management

The hair must be released as soon as possible. Cut or unwind the hair; however, be very careful that you do not only remove part of the hair or just one of several hairs. If, after an hour or so of observation, you are unsure that you have successfully released the hair, refer for general anaesthesia, where an incision may have to be made, down to the bone.

HAEMATOMAS AND CONTUSIONS

Following blunt injury, a significant amount of bleeding may go on underneath the surface and may not be apparent for some days. Fortunately, children are less prone to stiffness of the affected muscles than adults, because they heal quicker and are more determined to mobilize early. However, if the area is large, or mobility is a problem, early access to ultrasound therapy can help soften the tissues.

Management

Simple initial management of contused areas involves elevation of the affected part, if possible, and the application of ice packs (avoiding direct contact of the ice on the skin) at regular intervals for the first 24 hours, leaving them on for 20 minutes at a time.

BRUISING

Bruising is common in children and normally affects the lower limbs. The age of a bruise is more difficult to determine than is commonly thought. This has implications when considering non-accidental injury, if injuries are thought to have occurred at different times.

⚠ Always assess whether bruising is compatible with the history given, and refer for a second opinion if unsure (see Chapter 15 'Non-accidental Injury').

If there are multiple bruises, consider checking the platelet count and a clotting screen.

SPRAINS

A sprain is a soft tissue injury, such as tearing of a ligament. Children have stretchy tissues so are less prone to sprains than adults and generally recover much quicker.

⚠ Do not assume a simple sprain in toddlers and young children, since an underlying fracture is more likely.

General sprain management

The management of a sprain is similar to a contusion (see above). Early mobilization should be encouraged. Most emergency departments have advice sheets for common sprains, such as the ankle, shoulder or knee.

The mnemonic 'RICE' is often used: rest, ice, compression, and elevation. However, most children are reluctant to rest, and there is little evidence that more than 24 hours of rest is beneficial. Also, children often find using crutches difficult. Ice packs should be applied for 20 minutes, every 4 hours or so. Direct contact of ice with skin should be avoided, and packets of frozen peas are the a practical choice for most households! A compression bandage may help reduce swelling but does not provide support or improve healing.

Refer to the following chapters for specific sprains: neck, Chapter 6; knee and ankle, Chapter 10.

COMPARTMENT SYNDROME

In certain areas of the body, particularly the forearm and calf, the muscles are grouped together in compartments, separated by fascia. Following injury, swelling occurs and can be accommodated to an extent. However, as the pressure inside the compartment rises, the blood supply via the arterioles becomes jeopardized, and the muscles become ischaemic. A vicious cycle develops, which can result in necrosis, rhabdomyolysis, contractures and even loss of limb.

History

Early symptoms are pain and paraesthesia a few hours after injury.

Examination

Pulses often remain present until late on in the process. Passive stretching of the muscles is extremely painful and the limb may appear swollen.

Management

If in doubt, the pressure inside the compartment can be measured using a needle and transducer (pressures above 30 mmHg are worrying).

 An urgent surgical opinion is necessary for suspected compartment syndrome. Fasciotomy may be required.

DEGLOVING INJURIES

Degloving injuries occur when the skin and its blood supply are avulsed. This occurs with a blunt, shearing, mechanism of injury and may not be initially apparent, particularly if no laceration of the skin has occurred.

History

Areas prone to this kind of injury are the scalp, lower leg and foot. A typical mechanism of injury would be a car wheel running over the leg.

Examination

The skin is often contused and may be mobile. Swelling and/or an underlying fracture need not necessarily be present.

Management

Initial management consists of elevation of the limb or compression for a scalp laceration. A plastic surgeon must be involved, often jointly with an orthopaedic surgeon, since microsurgery, external fixation of fractures, fasciotomy or skin grafting may be necessary.

SKIN ABSCESSES

An abscess is a contained infection, which may be caused by a breach of the skin, an infected hair follicle or often for no obvious reason. They are relatively uncommon in children and the presence of a foreign body should be considered.

Once pus has collected, it cannot be treated successfully with antibiotics, but requires incision and drainage. The abscess may be quite deep seated and require general anaesthesia to achieve enough analgesia to allow full evacuation of its contents. Axillary, perianal and facial abscesses should be referred to a surgeon.

For straightforward abscesses, incision and drainage can be performed in the emergency department. This is best achieved with infiltration of local anaesthesia, and a large incision made to allow the pus out and to continue drainage. A non-adhesive dressing should be applied and the patient reviewed by their general practitioner.

Head and facial injuries

INTRODUCTION

(STOP) **Serious head injury is one of the commonest causes of death in children.**

Around half a million children per year present to the emergency department with head injury. Most of these are trivial, but head injury is one of the commonest causes of death in children. For the purposes of this book, a minor head injury is defined as one where the Glasgow Coma Score (GCS) is *normal*, i.e. the child is alert and orientated.

In infants and toddlers, the head is large compared with the rest of the body: therefore, they often fall head first. Injury severity correlates with the distance fallen. Non-mobile infants may fall from a height such as parents' arms, a bed or a baby chair put on a work surface. Skull fractures are relatively common in these cases, whereas injuries in toddlers tend to be caused by tripping over and are generally benign.

⚠ Think non-accidental injury in young children – is the history for this injury satisfactory? (See Chapter 15.)

⚠ Think of associated cervical spine injuries (see Chapter 6).

ASSESSMENT OF HEAD INJURIES

In children with a normal GCS, there is no clear correlation of intracranial injury with particular symptoms or the degree of the symptoms (such as number of vomiting episodes). However, relevant facts to elicit when taking history are:

• time of injury;
• mechanism of injury;
• loss of consciousness (LOC);
• seizure post-injury;
• memory of events during, and before and after injury;
• confusion;
• drowsiness;
• headache;
• vomiting.

Any injury that resulted in LOC more than a few seconds, a seizure, pre- or post-traumatic amnesia, confusion or vomiting more than twice is *not a minor injury*. However, short-term drowsiness, and vomiting once or twice are common symptoms, which do not generally require further investigation or hospital admission.

A minor head injury in some toddlers can trigger a *breath-holding attack,* which must be distinguished from loss of consciousness as a result of brain injury. The diagnosis is based on a careful history of a brief interval of consciousness and fright, before apnoea, and sometimes unconsciousness. The child recovers back to normal within a minute or so. There may have been previous similar episodes, such as after immunizations. Though frightening, it is an entirely benign phenomenon.

On examination, it is important to record the following:

• scalp signs;
• alertness, behaviour and GCS (in verbal children);
• pupil reactions and eye movements.

In non-verbal children it is sufficient to describe behaviour in narrative, such as 'playing happily' or 'quiet but interactive'. This is clearer to the reader than most paediatric versions of the GCS. Scalp signs may include lacerations or haematomas. Small, firm haematomas are generally benign, even if quite prominent. Larger, 'boggy' haematomas are highly indicative of underlying fracture, particularly in children under 1 year.

MANAGEMENT OF HEAD INJURIES

Local policies will, for the large part, determine your management. By the time children have arrived in the emergency department, been observed in the play area while waiting to be seen, then undergone a simple clinical assessment, the vast majority can be sent home with advice.

The role of X-rays and CT

In practice, there is a great deal of variation between hospitals and between individual doctors. Guidelines can be complex to draw up, particularly because the literature is confusing. For example, the definition of a 'minor' head injury, or the many studies of retrospective casenote reviews, in which the subtleties of behaviour are unlikely to have been recorded. Those children with worrisome findings on history or examination should at least be observed in hospital for a few hours. The correlation between skull fracture and intracranial bleeding is less clear than in adults, and particularly so in the shaken baby syndrome (see Chapter 15 'Non-accidental Injury'), so there is an argument that skull X-rays (SXRs) are largely redundant if there is access to a computed tomography (CT) scanner and there is cause for concern.

A SXR remains useful for several reasons, however. In a well child it can provide extra information without resorting to CT, which carries a high radiation dose and may require sedation. SXR is a useful screening tool for depressed fracture, if suspected by the mechanism of injury. Also, infants under 1 year are at increased risk of fracture because they have thin skulls, have poorly developed protective reflexes when they fall and are more at risk of non-accidental injury (NAI); at this age, head-injury related symptoms are vague and clinical examination difficult.

⚠️ If you perform a skull X-ray, treat it only as an additional piece of information and do not be falsely reassured if it is normal.

⚠️ Consult an anaesthetist or senior emergency department doctor for advice if the child may require sedation for a CT scan.

Table 5.1 provides some guidance about imaging, but use this in conjunction with your local head injury policy.

Table 5.1 Management of head injuries according to symptoms and signs.

Sign/symptom	Investigation	Admit/observation[a]
Penetrating injury	CT	√
GCS < 15	CT	√
Focal neurology	CT	√
History of LOC	CT if more than a minute or two	√
Vomited > twice	CT if persistent or other symptoms present	√
?NAI	CT	√
Persistent drowsiness	CT	√
Intoxicated	? CT Depends on mechanism of injury/scalp, limb or pupil signs/failure of improvement of GCS. Seek senior advice	√
?Depressed fracture	CT if high suspicion; SXR as screening tool if low suspicion	
?Base of skull fracture	CT if bleeding from nose or ear without local trauma. Other signs often take a few hours to appear	√
Boggy swelling	CT if high suspicion of fracture or other symptoms	
Non-walking infant	CT if significant mechanism or other symptoms, SXR as screening tool if well	
Around bedtime	Often appropriate	

[a]Observation for regular recording of drowsiness, confusion (GCS), abnormal behaviour or vomiting.

CT, computed tomography; GCS, Glasgow Coma Score; LOC, loss of consciousness; NAI, non-accidental injury; SXR, skull X-ray.

When do you consult a neurosurgeon?

This will depend on local guidelines. All children with a fracture should ideally undergo CT scan. Transfer under the care of neurosurgery is usually reserved for children with an abnormal brain on CT scan, after consultation.

Interpreting a skull X-ray

⚠ Brain injury can occur without skull vault fracture and *vice versa*.

See above. The standard views for visualization of skull fractures are the anteroposterior (A-P), lateral and Towne's view.

Fractures can be difficult to identify on X-rays. Features that make a lucent line more likely to be a fracture than a suture line or vascular marking are:

- sharply demarcated with uniform width throughout its length – does not taper or fork;
- does not fit with expected anatomy of suture lines;
- crosses a suture line;
- straight line;
- matches site of injury;
- does not correlate with a similar line on the opposite side of the skull (Figure 5.1).

Non-accidental injury (see also Chapter 15)

The following factors should alert you to the possibility of non-accidental head trauma (Figure 5.2):

- age under 2 years;
- head injury in a non-walking infant (check details of history);
- other unexplained injuries (all children must be examined fully if there is any concern);
- fracture or intracranial injury without history of significant trauma;
- 'growing' fracture (fracture > 3 mm and expanding), or fractures that are multiple, complex, branched or cross suture lines.

 If NAI suspected, refer to a senior doctor and your local child protection policy.

⚠ Fundoscopy is important, to examine for retinal haemorrhages.

Discharge instructions

Children must be watched by a competent adult for the next few hours, and brought back to the emergency department if they become drowsy, vomit more than once or if the carer is worried (saying that this means if the child is 'not himself or herself' is better than any head injury advice leaflet). For infants, the criteria for returning should be kept broad, and include poor feeding, drowsiness or persistent crying.

Parents of older children and teenagers should be advised that headache

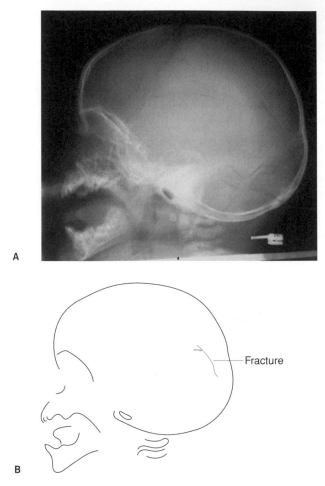

A

B

Figure 5.1 A linear parietal skull fracture.

is a common symptom post-head injury, and may continue for a week or two. They should only be concerned if it is severe, unresponsive to analgesia or associated with drowsiness, change in behaviour, vomiting or confusion. Other symptoms, such as dizziness, poor concentration and memory, blurred vision and tiredness are also very common, and can be explained to parents as 'concussion'.

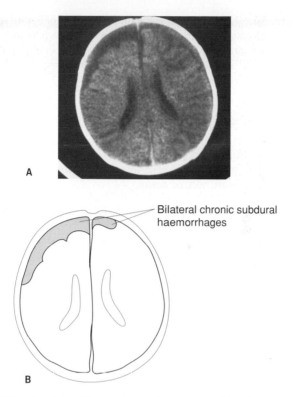

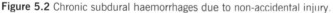
Bilateral chronic subdural haemorrhages

Figure 5.2 Chronic subdural haemorrhages due to non-accidental injury.

SCALP LACERATIONS

The scalp has a proliferate vascular supply, so parents can become very alarmed by small wounds. Most wounds will have stopped bleeding within 10 minutes but, if not, the use of lignocaine with adrenaline may facilitate suturing. Arterial 'spurters' may occur and are initially controlled by pressure bandaging. After insertion of large sutures through all the layers, the wound will tamponade itself.

⚠ Large lacerations may be a source of significant blood loss. This may be concealed if the child is supine and if the head is bandaged.

Larger lacerations should be explored with a sterile finger before suturing: a fracture may be palpable, although a defect in the galea may feel the same. Non-absorbable sutures should be removed after 5–7 days, but the use of absorbable sutures is better in children. If there is no tension on the wound, tissue adhesive glue is useful.

FACIAL LACERATIONS

Facial lacerations may bleed profusely. This rich blood supply means that wounds generally heal quickly, and infection is unusual, even in bites. However, facial scars are noticed easily.

⚠ If you lack confidence in ensuring a cosmetic repair for difficult areas, seek help.

Senior emergency department staff, orofaciomaxillary (OFM) and plastic surgeons are always happy to be referred difficult facial wounds in children.

🛑 Read the following sections in conjunction with Chapter 4 'Wounds and Soft Tissue Injuries'.

Scarring is affected by many things. An understanding of factors such as tension across a wound, or the special areas outlined below, is necessary when deciding your management. Suturing of faces is traumatic for most children, and it may be necessary to use *conscious sedation* (see Chapter 3 'Pain Management') or to refer for repair under general anaesthesia. Forehead wounds may bruise in the coming days, and track down to give 'black eyes'. It is worth warning parents about this innocent complication.

Eyelid wounds

⚠ Any wound involving the eyelid should be referred to an ophthalmologist.

Eyebrow wounds

Wounds involving the eyebrow require perfect anatomical repair with sutures, in order to avoid a *'step'* in the line of the eyebrow, which has significant cosmetic consequences. Despite accurate initial repair, a step can develop later as the child grows, so parents should be warned about this.

EYE INJURIES AND ORBITAL FRACTURES

You should be familiar with the use of a slit lamp and be able to test visual acuity. A modified Snellen's chart, using pictures, is available for younger children.

⚠ **Visual acuity must always be documented for eye injuries.**

Topical anaesthetic, e.g. benoxinate or proxymetacaine, is often necessary to facilitate thorough examination, and is effective almost instantly. The duration of action is usually 20 minutes or so, so that protection with a *patch* is unnecessary. However, photophobia is commonly present, and a feeling of direct pressure can be comforting, so a patch may be offered to older children. Patients often request anaesthetic drops to take home, because of the instant relief of symptoms, but this is not advisable because of the risk of secondary injury.

Many painful eyes cause blepharospasm and spasm of the ciliary apparatus. Administration of *mydriatic drops*, e.g. cyclopentolate, can relieve this but are best avoided in young children, since they may cause systemic anticholinergic effects.

For any breach of the corneal surface, *topical antibiotics*, e.g. chloramphenicol, should be prescribed for prevention of secondary infection until the patient is asymptomatic. Ointment can be administered twice daily, whereas drops require application every 3 hours; so, although it affects vision, if is often easier to administer ointment in children.

Corneal abrasions

History
Corneal abrasions may be very painful, or may present with a foreign body sensation (the foreign body may have been dislodged, leaving only an abrasion). Photophobia, watering and injection of the conjunctiva are usually present. There is often a history of the eye being scratched, e.g. by a zip or twig. It is worth looking for a corneal abrasion in a persistently crying baby (these abrasions are often sustained during nappy changing).

Examination
Abrasions are easier to see with fluorescein staining. It is not necessary for a child to cooperate with slit-lamp examination: shining a blue or green light (e.g. using an ophthalmoscope) from a distance is less threatening.

Management
Abrasions can be managed by covering with an eye patch (see above) and prescription of antibiotic ointment to prevent secondary infection. Abrasions smaller than the size of the pupil, and not crossing the pupil, do not require follow-up.

Corneal foreign bodies

History
Small foreign bodies (FBs) may enter the eye while working with tools, or simply when carried by the wind. However, there is usually a history of acute onset of symptoms.

Examination
Using a cotton-wool bud, with the patient looking downwards, evert the upper eyelid in case the FB is trapped underneath. Anaesthetic drops may be needed. If no FB is found, use a slit lamp wherever possible, to check the cornea. If still unsuccessful, consider an abrasion (instil fluorescein drops) or an allergic reaction (particularly if the FB was organic).

Management
For removal of corneal foreign bodies see Chapter 17 'Practical Procedures'. Orbital X-rays are not needed unless a high-velocity mechanism of injury, e.g. chiselling or high-pressure jets, is given. After removal, apply a patch and prescribe antibiotic ointment (see above), and arrange follow-up.

Chemical injuries

If possible, differentiate between acid and alkaline liquids using litmus paper.

⚠ Different types of litmus paper are available. Use the paper that gives you a pH value.

⚠ Litmus paper is not useful for monitoring response to irrigation, unless tested half an hour after irrigation has stopped and the child is symptom free.

Acids
Children commonly get acidic liquids in their eyes, e.g. household cleaning fluids. If the fluid is acidic, then irrigation using 500 ml of saline, via an IV giving set, should suffice. Most injuries are superficial because acids cause coagulation of the surface tissues, thus forming a protective barrier to further damage. No follow-up is necessary unless they remain symptomatic.

Alkalis

⚠ Alkaline injuries are much more serious than acid injuries.

Alkalis are found in household cleaning products, and may be highly concentrated in substances, such as oven cleaner or dishwasher tablets. Wet concrete is also alkaline and, while uncommon as a childhood injury, is very serious.

Alkalis permeate between cell membranes, causing deep-seated damage. Deceptively, they may be less painful than acids initially. Irrigate immediately (as above) with large volumes and seek advice from an ophthalmologist. Some need hospital admission for constant irrigation.

'Blow-out' fracture of the inferior orbital margin

History
This injury occurs when an object, e.g. a small ball, hits the eye rather than the zygoma. The contents of the orbit are pushed down through the orbital floor, since this is the weakest point. There may be an associated hyphaema (see below).

Examination
The inferior rectus muscle becomes trapped, causing diplopia on upward gaze. Enophthalmos may occur. The classical appearance on X-ray is the ball of proptosed tissue, described as a 'teardrop' visible in the maxillary antrum (see Figure 5.3).

Management
All 'blow-out' fractures must be discussed with an ophthalmologist immediately. It is crucial that the child does not blow their nose: this can severely worsen the entrapment of soft tissues.

Hyphaema

History
A hyphaema occurs when the eye is struck and bleeding occurs into the anterior chamber.

Examination
There is photophobia and a fluid level may be visible in front of the iris, but it may require a slit lamp for detection.

Management
The child should be persuaded to rest, in order to prevent extension of the bleed. Secondary haemorrhage may cause acute glaucoma or corneal

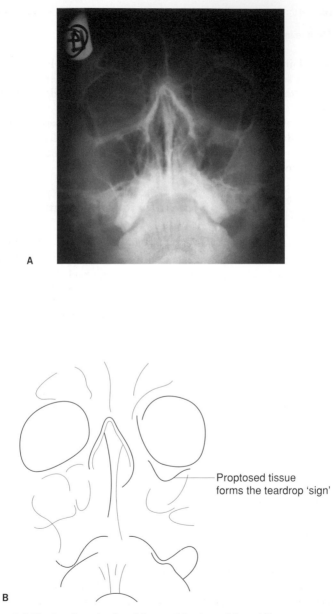

A

B

Proptosed tissue
forms the teardrop 'sign'

Figure 5.3 The teardrop sign in a 'blow-out' fracture of the orbit.

staining. Hospital admission may be required. Refer to an ophthalmologist immediately.

Penetrating injuries of the globe

⚠ All penetrating injuries must be referred to an ophthalmologist immediately.

Signs may be subtle – look for abnormal pupil shape or reaction, decreased acuity and vitreous extrusion.

INJURIES OF THE EAR

The pinna

Wounds involving the *cartilage* should be referred to orofaciomaxillary (OFM), or ear, nose and throat (ENT) surgeons. A blow to the pinna may cause a *haematoma*. If this becomes tense, necrosis of the inner cartilage may occur, causing lifelong deformity ('cauliflower ears'). If tense, consult an ENT surgeon for drainage; if not, apply a pressure bandage using a gauze pack and a 'turban' bandage, and arrange review the following day.

The tympanic membrane

This may perforate following a blow to the side of the head, but more typically following foreign body insertion, particularly cotton-wool buds. Examination may be difficult because of pain. Spontaneous healing usually occurs, but the child should avoid swimming and be examined by their general practitioner after 3–4 weeks to ensure healing has occurred.

NASAL INJURIES

Nasal fractures

History
A direct blow to the nose may result in fracture. This is less likely in young children because the nasal bone is not calcified. It is not necessary to X-ray for nasal fractures, as the management is symptomatic and/or cosmetic.

Examination

⚠ **Always examine specifically for a septal haematoma.**

Record displacement of the nose, and always document the presence or absence of a septal haematoma, which looks like a dark, bulging mass. A similar process as happens in the pinna can occur (see above), resulting in a 'saddle nose' deformity. If present, refer to ENT immediately for drainage.

Management

Advise the patient that the swelling will increase over the next few days and they may develop 'black eyes'. The only treatment is to apply ice packs in the first 24 hours. Find out your local arrangements for follow-up in an outpatient ENT clinic in 5–10 days' time. The purpose of follow-up is for consideration of manipulation of the fracture, if there is deformity or nasal obstruction. This is impossible to assess in the first few days, hence the delay. Follow-up is not necessary if the nose is clearly not displaced.

ORAL INJURIES

Injuries of the mouth area are common. Fortunately they heal well, but there are a few pitfalls.

Lacerations crossing the vermillion border of the lip

Wounds crossing the vermillion border of the lip require perfect anatomical repair with sutures, to avoid a '*step*' in the line of lip border, which has greater cosmetic consequences for this part of the body than for most others (except the eyebrow). Despite accurate initial repair, a step may develop later, as the child grows. Parents should be warned about this.

'Through and through' lacerations of the lip

This means that the wound extends from the inside of the mouth to the skin outside, and is usually caused by the teeth. Careful repair with sutures is necessary to avoid cosmetic deformity, accumulation of food in the tract or formation of a sinus. A layered repair may be necessary: do not attempt this yourself if you are unsure you have the necessary skills.

Torn frenulum

The frenulum attaches the upper lip to the gum, between the two first incisors. It contains a small artery, which bleeds profusely initially, then usually goes into spasm and stops, particularly if cold compresses and pressure are applied. Suturing is rarely necessary.

⚠ Check the history. This injury is caused by a direct blow to the upper lip, which may occur as a result of non-accidental injury.

Wounds of the buccal cavity

Most wounds heal quickly by themselves. Sutures are only necessary if they are gaping, or a piece of tissue will interfere with chewing. Use absorbable materials if sutures are necessary. For this, conscious sedation or general anaesthesia is usually necessary. Ice lollipops can help with pain. Advise soft diet, avoiding foods such as potato crisps for a few days. Broad-spectrum antibiotics, e.g. co-amoxyclavulinic acid, are frequently prescribed. Warn the parents that the wound will look yellow in the next couple of days.

Lacerations of the tongue

The same principles apply as for wounds of the buccal cavity (see above).

Penetrating intra-oral injuries

This type of injury commonly occurs if a child trips while holding something in their mouths. It is important to recognize if the object may have penetrated through the palate (usually soft palate). A small wound may hide a significant injury, which may result in a retropharyngeal abscess and mediastinitis. If in doubt, request a lateral soft tissue X-ray of the neck and refer to ENT.

⚠ Failure to recognize perforation of the palate may result in severe illness, and even death.

DENTAL INJURIES

The most important consideration in dental injuries is whether the tooth is a deciduous or permanent tooth. In general, injuries to deciduous teeth can be reviewed by a dentist the following day, although an avulsed tooth is worth reimplanting (as below), if possible.

Avulsion of a tooth

⚠ Avulsion of a permanent tooth is an emergency – the tooth should be reimplanted within minutes if possible.

When a permanent tooth is avulsed, the root starts to die within half an hour, so that reimplantation rapidly becomes unsuccessful, or if the tooth reattaches it may become discoloured. A simple first-aid measure is to keep the tooth in the mouth (saliva is protective) or in a cup of milk, pending reimplantation.

As soon as possible, the tooth should be reimplanted into the socket and held in position by the child (by occluding the mouth or with a finger) or by an adult, until an OFM doctor can come and fix it in position.

Wobbly or chipped teeth

Most of these injuries can be seen by the patient's own dentist, the next working day. Where there is either suspicion of alveolar fracture, or significant difficulty with occlusion, discuss with the OFM service.

CHIN LACERATIONS

Wounds under the chin occur frequently, when children fall forwards or come off a bicycle. They can nearly always be repaired with adhesive strips, even if they are gaping. Assess for mandibular fracture (below).

FRACTURES OF THE MANDIBLE

History

These are uncommon in children and occur most often with a fall on to the point of the chin (Figure 5.4). They may be caused by a punch in adolescents. Remember that the mandible is a ring-type structure, so it may fracture in two places, even with one point of impact, e.g. fracture of the body with associated fracture of the condylar neck.

Examination

The hallmarks of mandibular fracture are pain, swelling, malocclusion, poor opening (except crack fractures of the condylar neck) and bruising

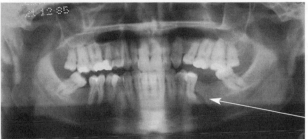

Fracture

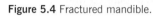

Figure 5.4 Fractured mandible.

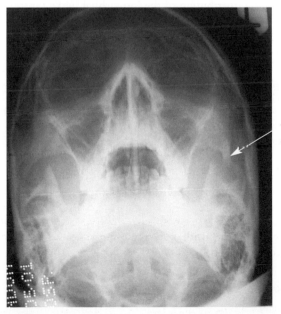

Displaced fracture of zygoma

Figure 5.5 Fractured left zygoma.

(particularly around the gum or sublingually). There may be anaesthesia in the distribution of a mental nerve.

Management

Refer all fractures to the OFM service.

FRACTURES OF THE ZYGOMATIC COMPLEX

History

Fractures of the zygoma are also unusual in children, and usually associated with quite severe injury or a punch (Figure 5.5).

Examination

The hallmark signs of zygomatic fracture are unilateral epistaxis, swelling and bruising of the area (which may include the eyelids), subconjunctival haemorrhage (the posterior border of which can not be seen) and reduced sensation in the distribution of the infraorbital nerve (around the cheek, nose, gum and lip on the affected side). Other signs, which are mentioned in textbooks, are more apparent later, such as flattening of the contour of the cheek, and a palpable step in the orbital margin.

Management

In this age group, it is best to ask advice, the same day, from the OFM service.

Neck and back injuries

INTRODUCTION

Spinal injuries are rare in children and usually associated with injury mechanisms such as being knocked down by a car or trampolining accidents. Although serious injury is rare, minor injury to the neck and back is common, and it is important to feel secure in assessing severity.

🛑 **If major trauma – resuscitate A B C first, with neck immobilized. See APLS guidelines.**

Children may sustain fractures and/or dislocations of the spine, which may or may not be stable, or associated with cord injury. A history of transient neurological symptoms, such as numbness or tingling (seconds or minutes) is not uncommon, and usually indicates minor cord contusion.

In the cervical spine, it is not uncommon for children to sustain cord injury without fracture, as a result of ligamentous injury. In fact, immediately following impact, the ligaments can return to their normal position, making diagnosis very difficult. Plain films may appear normal, and the injury is only visible on CT or magnetic resonance imaging (MRI) scan. If cord injury is present, this may be called 'SCIWORA': Spinal Cord Injury Without Radiographic Abnormality.

Thoracic and lumbar fractures are also rare in childhood. Typical mechanisms would include falling from a height or a vehicle crash without an appropriate seat belt.

WHAT IS SPINAL IMMOBILIZATION?

Cervical spinal immobilization consists of the following:
1 A hard collar, which restricts flexion, extension and some lateral movement. It should be sized according to the manufacturer's guidelines.
2 Specially designed head blocks/sandbags/bags of IV fluids, either side of the neck, to prevent lateral movements.
3 Tape or straps across the forehead and chin, to discourage rotational movement (Figure 6.1).

Or

Another person holding the head in line with the body, in the neutral position, preventing any head movements (Figures 6.2 and 6.3).

The child may arrive on a long, rigid, spinal board (Figure 6.4), which prevents movement of the thoracic and lumbar spine. This is an extrication device, which is used, in the pre-hospital phase. The child should be log-rolled off this hard board and allowed to lie on a firm stretcher (see Chapter 17 'Practical Procedures').

Alternative devices include a 'scoop' bivalve stretcher (Figure 6.5); this undoes at the top and the bottom, thus avoiding the need for log-rolling. Another option is a vacuum mattress, which fits around the child better, and can be deflated to allow access to the child, then reinflated for transfers.

SHOULD I IMMOBILIZE THE CHILD?

Common sense needs to be applied. Immobilization is disorientating, uncomfortable and upsets children, making the rest of the examination

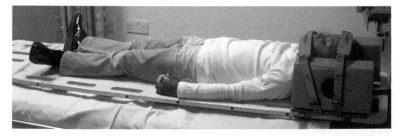

Figure 6.1 Child on long spinal board, with straps and blocks supplementing hard cervical collar.

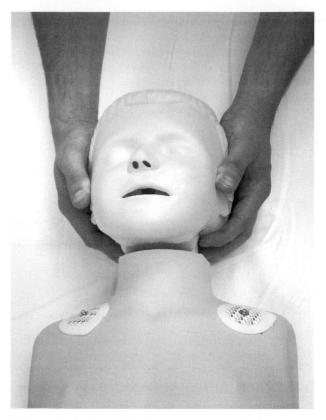

Figure 6.2 Manual in-line immobilization of the cervical spine from above.

difficult. If the child is very agitated and spinal precautions are necessary, immobilization may be harmful, as the body is pivoting on the neck. Either use manual immobilization (e.g. parent) or allow the child to move, retaining the hard collar, if possible, for some protection.

For mechanisms such as those described in the introduction to this chapter it is wise to immobilize all children. Those brought by ambulance will frequently have been immobilized already. This need not be continued if further assessment is normal (see below).

Children who present more than a few hours since the injury or who are happily walking around, do not need full spinal immobilization. Even if ligamentous or bony injury is present, it is likely to be stable.

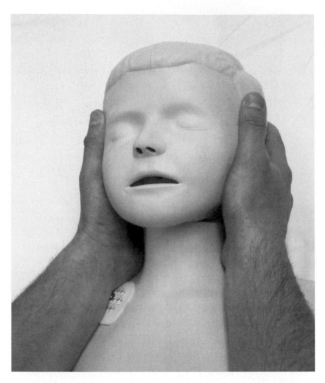

Figure 6.3 Manual in-line immobilization of the cervical spine from below.

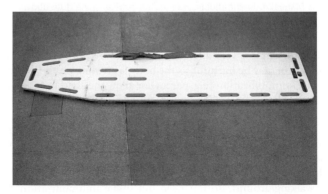

Figure 6.4 Long spinal board.

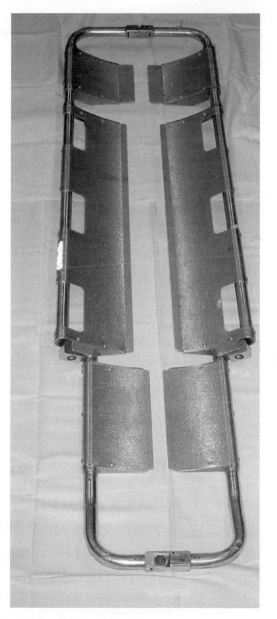

Figure 6.5 Bivalve stretcher.

Holding the head in a particular position, or torticollis, may imply significant injury (see below). However, children exhibiting this posture should not be forced to lie down in a neutral position, as this may do further harm.

CLINICALLY CLEARING THE NECK

Look for torticollis (see above). Significant injury, such as unifacet dislocation, can be caused by apparently minor mechanisms, such as a 'clash of heads' or the head being hit by a football.

If the child is conscious and cooperative, ask if their neck or back hurts, then assess their neurology. If the neurology is normal, remove the collar, with an assistant holding the head (see above), then palpate for midline tenderness.

If any of the following are present, reimmobilization and imaging of the neck are required.
- clouding of consciousness, e.g. alcohol;
- distracting painful injury elsewhere;
- neurological symptoms or signs;
- torticollis or abnormal posture of head;
- midline tenderness.

If none of the above is present, it is reasonable to ask the child to try moving their neck side to side, and off the bed. **Do not** force them to move. If there is limitation of movement, proceed to X-ray.

If all the above features are normal, consider back injury, but if asymptomatic, allow the child to sit up and prescribe analgesia (see Chapter 3 'Pain Management'). If X-ray examination is required, those with normal films **and** no abnormal neurology can be freed up.

THE LOG-ROLL EXAMINATION OF THE THORACIC AND LUMBAR SPINE

If you suspect back injury, again examine the neurology first. To examine the back, perform a controlled log-roll ensuring the spine remains aligned (see Figures 6.6 and 6.7). Before attempting this, reassure the child that they do not need to 'help' or move, and that they will not fall off the side, because of the people holding them. Roll the child only as far as is necessary to inspect the back and palpate the whole spine for tenderness.

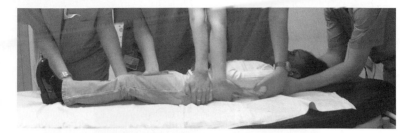

Figure 6.6 Hand positions for a log-roll.

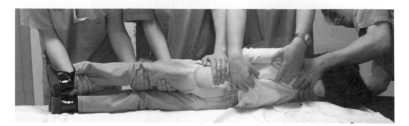

Figure 6.7 A log-roll.

X-RAYS

Interpretation of children's spine X-rays can be difficult even for the experienced. In younger children there is frequently pseudo-subluxation of C2 on C3 (Figure 6.8), or C3 on C4. In addition there are multiple physeal lines and ossification centres, such as the ring apophyses visible in puberty at the corners of vertebral bodies, which may be mistaken for teardrop fractures.

Indirect evidence of injury may be seen in cervical X-rays by assessing soft tissue swelling (Figure 6.9). If you detect a fracture, look for another as it is possible to find multiple levels involved in spinal injuries.

⚠️ If in doubt, continue immobilization until senior help is available.

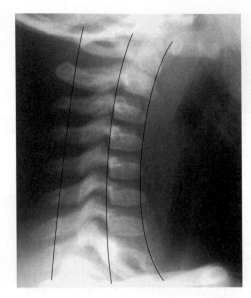

Figure 6.8 Pseudo-subluxation of C2 on C3. C2 appears to be slipped forwards on C3 by the normal rules of alignment. However, note normal alignment posteriorly.

CERVICAL SPINE INJURIES

A full description of possible cervical spine injuries is beyond the remit of this book.

Sprains

Neck sprains are reasonably common in children. They may occur on, or shortly after, waking up. Usually a reasonably good range of movement is present. The parents may be concerned about the possibility of meningitis. No imaging is necessary if there is no torticollis (see above) or history of injury. Treatment involves simple painkillers, ice packs (such as a packet of frozen peas held on the neck for 20 minutes, every 4 hours or so), and exercises to avoid stiffness.

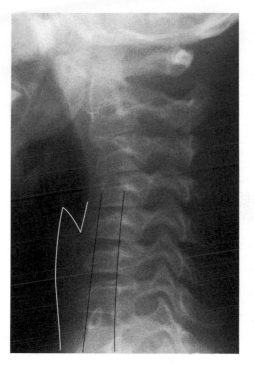

Figure 6.9 Apparent soft tissue swelling. The soft tissue shadow is wider than the width of the vertebral bodies. This can happen with crying or neck flexion, and does not always imply injury.

Fractures and dislocations

The upper three vertebrae are more commonly involved in younger children, as opposed to the lower cervical vertebrae and C7/T1 junction, which is a more common injury pattern in adolescents and adults. Unifacet dislocation of C1 or C2 may occur (see above). CT is required to make the diagnosis.

THORACIC AND LUMBAR SPINE INJURIES

Although spinal injuries are rare, the most common X-ray finding is anterior wedging of the vertebrae from forced flexion mechanisms of injury. CT is necessary to look for posterior protrusion of bone fragments.

Fractures and dislocations
– general approach

INTRODUCTION

Before the age of 16, around 50% of boys and 25% of girls will sustain a fracture. Dislocations, however, are very uncommon. The bones of children (Figure 7.1) differ from adults in three respects, as listed below.

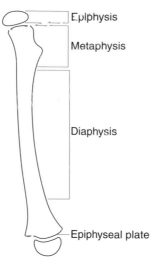

Epiphysis

Metaphysis

Diaphysis

Epiphyseal plate

Figure 7.1 A child's bone.

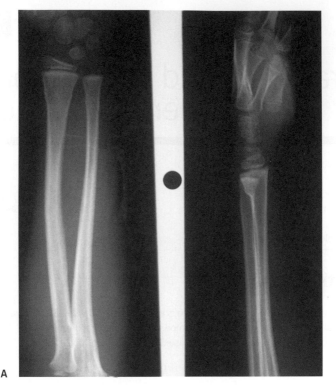

A

Figure 7.2 A torus fracture.

- A child's bone is less brittle than that of an adult owing to its higher collagen to bone ratio. Therefore, incomplete fractures may occur (torus or greenstick fractures).
- The growth plates, or epiphyses, may bear the brunt of the injury (Salter-Harris classification).
- The periosteum in young children is very strong, and protects the bone from fracture or can limit displacement if it does fracture, e.g. a 'toddler's' fracture of the tibia.

Torus fractures

This is when the cortex buckles with no apparent break. This is known as a torus or buckle fracture (Figure 7.2).

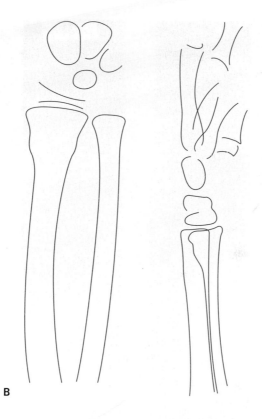

B

Greenstick fractures

In a greenstick fracture, one cortical surface breaks, while the opposite surface merely buckles (Figure 7.3). The periosteum, over the buckled bone, often remains intact.

Epiphyseal fractures

A child's bone must also have the ability to grow and it achieves this by the presence of epiphyseal growth plates. The epiphyseal plate is strong in small children, but becomes a relatively weak spot in middle childhood and various patterns of injuries can occur at this site. These injuries have been classified into five types – the Salter–Harris classification (Figure 7.4). The diagram demonstrates an easy way to memorize the five types. Type II is the most common injury.

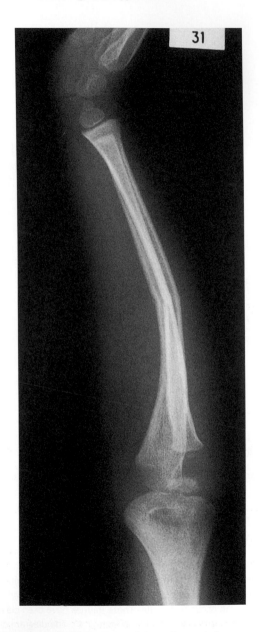

Figure 7.3 Midshaft greenstick fractures of the radius and ulna.

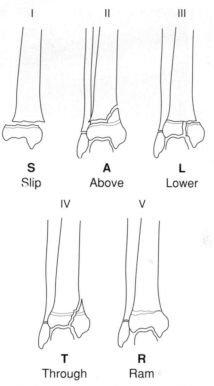

Figure 7.4 The Salter–Harris classification of epiphyseal injuries.

It is important that these injuries are identified and treated appropriately. Not only does the fracture need to heal, but also the child needs to continue with a normal growth pattern. The type V injury is very difficult to diagnose initially and may present as abnormal growth many months later.

Metaphyseal fractures

These fractures are almost pathognomonic of non-accidental injury (see Chapter 15) (Figure 7.5). They may be very subtle when acute, but the injury becomes more obvious as callus forms and a periosteal reaction occurs along the length of the metaphyseal cortex. This is seen when there is a delay in presentation, or a skeletal survey is done.

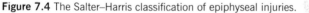

🛑 **If you see a metaphyseal fracture, call for senior help and refer to your local child protection policy.**

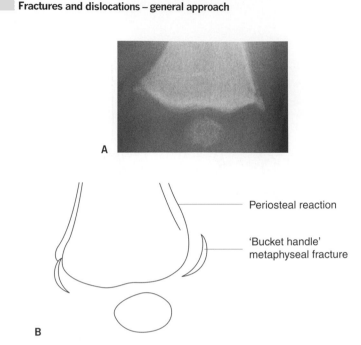

A

Periosteal reaction

'Bucket handle' metaphyseal fracture

B

Figure 7.5 Metaphyseal fracture characteristic of non-accidental injury

ASSESSMENT OF FRACTURES AND DISLOCATIONS

Mechanism of injury

The history of the mechanism of injury will provide the best clues as to the injuries sustained. For example, falling over is more likely to break a bone than banging against something.

⚠ **If significant force is involved, e.g. road traffic accident, assume major trauma until proven otherwise.**

A direct blow may cause a fracture and/or dislocation at that site. More often fractures occur as a result of indirect forces. For example, a fall on an outstretched hand may lead to a fractured distal radius, a supracondylar fracture of the elbow or a fractured clavicle.

⚠ **Is the history for this injury satisfactory? (See Chapter 15 'Non-accidental Injury'.)**

Examination

When examining for evidence of a fracture or dislocation, you should look, then feel, then very gently try to move the affected area, unless it is very painful.

Look for:
- deformity;
- swelling;
- bruising;
- abnormal posture or alignment;
- rotation;
- distribution and depth of open wounds.

Feel for:
- tenderness – try to localize this to the point of maximal tenderness;
- an obvious step;
- distal pulse/capillary refill/sensation.

The more localized the tenderness, the more likely there is a fracture present. If the child is unable to localize the pain, try asking them to press around and tell you where it hurts the most. If they are not very specific, you can then try gently pressing yourself, and offer options 'this bit or this bit?' or 'number one, number two or number three' as you try different areas. For pre-verbal children it may be difficult, but by being gentle and systematic, and sometimes repeating the pressing while the child is distracted, you can localize the injury.

Move: Attempt movement at the joint above and below the site of injury (**only** if pain allows). Allow the child active movements before attempting passive movements. Particularly in small children, the only abnormality may be loss of normal use of the limb. Give the child an opportunity to use the limb, e.g. introduce them to some toys and watch how the limb is held or used. Document how much the child is using the limb, and the range of movement (e.g. flexion, extension, supination, pronation, rotation).

X-RAYS

When to X-ray

If in doubt, have a low threshold for requesting X-rays. Young children, in particular, can have quite subtle signs for fractures, such as greenstick fractures. Most parents will be expecting you to X-ray their child, but you have to use your experience and explain the potential risks of radiation, if you consider the X-ray to be unnecessary.

To ensure adequate X-rays are taken, always give as much information as possible on the request card. The area you specify on your request should be as focused as possible (see Table 7.1 below). For midshaft longbone fractures, the joint above and the joint below should be seen. To diagnose and fully assess the injury, two films should be taken at right angles to each other: these are most usually anteroposterior and lateral views, but usually the radiographer will decide this for you.

Which X-rays to request

This is crucial, if you are not to miss fractures. If in doubt, ask a radiographer for his or her advice, explaining the context. The view that you request is crucial in ensuring you do not miss the fracture (see Table 7.1).

Interpretation of paediatric X-rays

Interpreting paediatric X-rays comes with practice. Fractures may be very subtle and the presence of various ossification centres around joints can add to the confusion. If in doubt about an X-ray, always seek a second opinion. It is important to note any significant angulation (greater than 20°) or dis-

Table 7.1 Requests for radiographic studies.

Body area	Appropriate request	Injury or fracture (#) suspected
Upper limb	Shoulder	Ruptured acromio-clavicular joint or dislocation head of humerus
	Clavicle	# clavicle
	Humerus	# shaft humerus
	Elbow	Supracondylar #, # epicondyle, # radial head or neck, # olecranon
	Forearm	# shaft radius / ulna
	Wrist	# distal radius / ulna
	Scaphoid views	# or dislocation of any carpal bones
	Hand	# metacarpals
	Fingers / thumb	# or dislocation phalanges or joints
Lower limb	Femur	# femur
	Knee	Dislocated or # patella, #s of knee itself
	Tibia and fibula	# tibia or fibula
	Ankle	# medial or lateral malleolus, or distal tibia
	Foot	All bones of foot, except calcaneum
	Calcaneum	Calcaneum
Spine	Peg view	Odontoid peg and C1
	Lateral cervical spine	C1 – T1
	Anteroposterior C spine	C1 – T1
	Thoracic	
	Lumbar	

placement (greater than 50%) of the distal fragment of a fracture when reviewing the X-ray.

PRINCIPLES OF MANAGEMENT

⚠ Major trauma – resuscitate A B C. See APLS guidelines.

⚠ If NAI is suspected, refer to both orthopaedic and paediatric teams.

General principles

Management of pain is paramount. Appropriate pain relief should be offered (see Chapter 3 'Pain Management'). Immobilizing a fracture, whether with splint, plaster cast or sling, will dramatically improve pain. Similarly, reduction of a dislocation provides dramatic pain relief, but should not be attempted without appropriate analgesia, sedation or anaesthesia, as required for the procedure.

Simple fractures, with no axial rotation, and only minor degrees of angulation and displacement will simply require a plaster cast and orthopaedic clinic follow-up.

Compound fractures

Compound fractures need to be thoroughly cleaned under operating theatre conditions as soon as possible after injury. Fracture management may also vary considerably from a similar non-compound fracture.

⚠ Suspect a compound fracture if there is any kind of wound overlying, or near to, the fracture. Call for orthopaedic assistance immediately.

If you suspect a compound fracture, dress the wound with an antiseptic-soaked dressing, and give parenteral anti-staphylococcal antibiotics. Prevent other people from continually disturbing the wound. A Polaroid™ or digital camera can be invaluable in this situation.

Closed fractures

Most fractures require immobilization in a plaster cast, both for healing and for pain management. Manipulation under anaesthetic/sedation (MUA) or internal fixation, are usually required for the following:

Fractures:
- significant clinical deformity;
- axial rotation;
- significant angulation (usually greater than 20°);
- significant displacement.

Dislocations – all dislocations.
Immediate referral to orthopaedics is required for the following:
- fracture or dislocation requiring general anaesthetic for MUA (see above);
- traction in hospital;
- risk of compartment syndrome (see Chapter 4 'Wounds and Soft Tissue Injuries');
- evidence of neurological or vascular compromise.

If you are sending the child home, ensure the family has analgesia (see Chapter 3 'Pain Management') and are encouraged to give it.

Advice regarding plaster casts

If a plaster cast has been applied, ensure that the family knows it should not get wet. They must also understand to return if the plaster is uncomfortable or painful, if the limb becomes swollen or if there is coldness, tingling or numbness distally.

Injuries of the upper limb

INTRODUCTION

For general principles of assessment, investigation and management of fractures and dislocations in children, see Chapter 7. Fractures of the upper limb are much more common than the lower limb. The most common fractures are of the distal radius and clavicle.

CLAVICLE FRACTURE

Assessment

Fracture of the clavicle usually occurs following a fall. It is common throughout childhood, with younger children tending to be less symptomatic. Birth injuries may present several weeks later. Toddlers may present a day or two after injury. While delay in presentation should normally ring 'alarm bells' (see Chapter 15 'Non-accidental Injury'), it is quite common with clavicular fractures. In young children focal tenderness may not occur and reasonable arm function may be preserved; however, abduction of the arm is usually painful. If the child can abduct beyond 90°, fracture is unlikely and X-rays are not needed. Occasionally, tenting of the skin over a displaced fracture occurs. This looks dramatic but does not need immediate referral.

X-ray (Figure 8.1)

Young children may have a greenstick fracture, which may be difficult to see because the clavicle curves.

Management

After appropriate analgesia, apply a broad arm sling, or collar and cuff (see Chapter 17 'Practical Procedures'), and arrange orthopaedic clinic

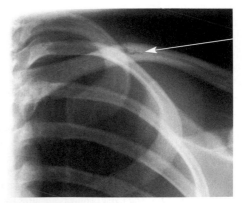

Subtle mid-claviclar greenstick fracture

Figure 8.1 Fractured clavicle.

follow-up. If a toddler will not keep a sling on, do not worry, simply reassure the parents that the bone will heal well. Advise all parents that a lump may be present after healing, which will reduce in size as the child grows.

SHOULDER DISLOCATION

Gleno-humeral dislocation is uncommon in children, and tends only to occur with severe force, in teenagers, during fits, or in those with connective tissue disorders.

Assessment

The deformity is usually obvious, and pain severe. There is a palpable step below the acromion. Do not attempt to move the arm. There may be associated sensory loss over the deltoid area owing to compression of the axillary nerve, which usually resolves once the joint is relocated.

Management

Analgesia is the priority (see Chapter 3 'Pain Management'). However the best analgesia is reduction of the dislocation. An X-ray should be performed first, though, to see if it is an anterior (>90%) or posterior dislocation, and whether there is an associated fracture (in which case orthopaedic referral is recommended).

X-ray (Figure 8.2)

Reduction of the dislocation depends on adequate muscle relaxation. Much of this can be achieved through psychological measures (Chapter 3), so sedation is not always necessary. Self-reduction is possible after analgesia, particularly if lying prone and in recurrent dislocations. There is no place for brute force, and none of the more complicated methods of reduction is a substitute for very slow, gentle traction (to avoid muscle spasm) followed by gentle abduction then external rotation, if necessary. On reduction a 'clunk' may or may not be felt, but the patient usually feels dramatically better and passive movement is restored.

After reduction, place the arm in a broad arm sling (see Chapter 17 'Practical Procedures') and X-ray again. Arrange follow-up within a few days.

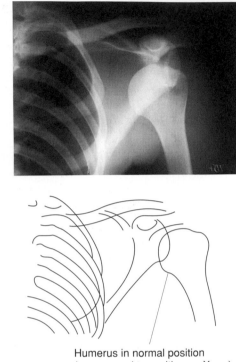

A

B Humerus in normal position
(as opposed to position on X-ray)

Figure 8.2 Dislocated shoulder.

ACROMIO-CLAVICULAR JOINT INJURY

Assessment

This usually occurs in teenagers following a fall directly on to the shoulder. Tenderness with or without swelling is usually localized to the point where the acromion meets the clavicle. Deformity may be seen if severe and may mimic gleno-humeral dislocation.

X-rays

These are necessary only if deformity is seen.

Management

Symptomatic management in a broad arm sling is nearly always sufficient. Arrange follow-up with orthopaedic clinics in the next few days for those with deformity. Advise that a persistent lump may occur.

PROXIMAL HUMERUS FRACTURE

Assessment

Fracture of the neck of the humerus can occur by falling on to the shoulder itself or on to the outstretched hand. Ability to abduct the arm beyond 90° makes a fracture unlikely.

X-ray (Figure 8.3)

X-ray findings may be subtle. Look for epiphyseal fracture or a buckle of the metaphysis.

Management

If the epiphyseal fracture is significantly displaced or there is angulation greater than 20°, refer immediately for orthopaedic opinion. Otherwise, apply a collar and cuff (see Chapter 17 'Practical Procedures') and arrange orthopaedic clinic follow-up.

HUMERAL SHAFT FRACTURE

Assessment

Fracture of the humeral shaft is uncommon. Clinical diagnosis is usually straightforward.

 A spiral fracture of the humerus is virtually pathognomonic of non-accidental injury (see Chapter 15).

Assess for radial nerve injury, looking for signs of wrist drop or sensory loss in the thumb web-space on the dorsum of the hand.

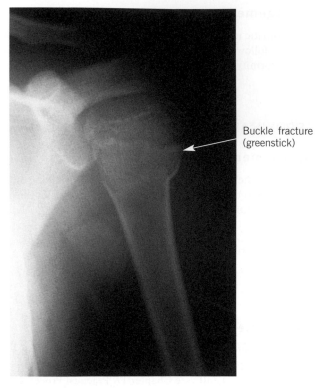

Buckle fracture
(greenstick)

Figure 8.3 Fractured neck of humerus.

X-ray (Figure 8.4)

Management

⚠ **For a spiral fracture, refer immediately to orthopaedics and invoke your local child protection policy.**

For fractures with neurological deficit or displacement, refer for an immediate orthopaedic opinion. The remainder should be placed in a collar and cuff (see Chapter 17, 'Practical Procedures'), and orthopaedic clinic follow-up arranged.

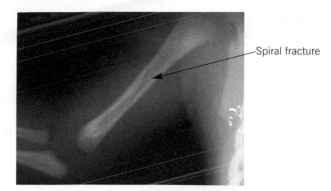

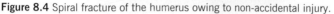

Figure 8.4 Spiral fracture of the humerus owing to non-accidental injury.

THE ELBOW – GENERAL

The many different ossification centres around the elbow make interpretation of children's X-rays particularly difficult. If in doubt, check a paediatric radiology textbook or consult a senior.

The presence of a joint effusion makes a fracture much more likely. On examination, swelling may be seen but this can be quite subtle. Position both the child's elbows at 90° and compare the dimples on each side. On X-ray, an effusion is detected by a positive 'fat pad sign' on the lateral view.

In a normal joint, fat lines the outside of the joint capsule and is visible anterior to the humerus on the lateral view because flexion makes it more prominent. It is seen as a small dark area (see Figure 8.5). When there is a

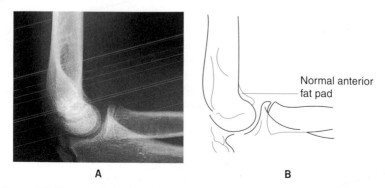

Figure 8.5 Normal anterior fat pad seen as a small lucency.

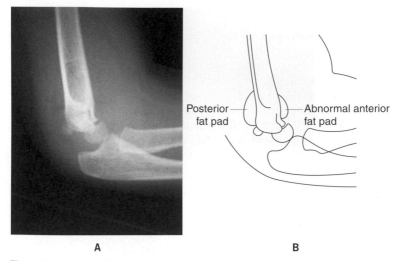

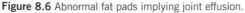

A   B

Figure 8.6 Abnormal fat pads implying joint effusion.

joint effusion, the anterior fat pad becomes elevated away from the humerus, and the normally flat (stretched) posterior fat pad becomes visible (see Figure 8.6).

The fat pad sign is strongly suggestive of an intra-articular fracture. However, the absence of a fat pad does not rule out a fracture. Use your clinical examination to guide your management.

SUPRACONDYLAR HUMERAL FRACTURE

Assessment

This a common fracture in children, with a peak age at about 8 years. It is generally caused by a fall. There is usually swelling (see above for detection), which may be mild or severe with deformity. It can be difficult to distinguish the more severe cases from a dislocated elbow (see below), although the management is similar.

It is extremely important to examine and record the distal neurological and vascular status of the arm. This fracture is associated with vascular compromise owing to impingement of the brachial artery by the distal humeral fragment or the associated haematoma. Signs vary from a pulseless, pale, painful forearm to more subtle changes in pulse volume or capillary refill.

X-ray

There is a wide range of possible X-ray findings. There may be a simple greenstick fracture, which may be difficult to detect, although a joint effusion is usually present. At the opposite extreme, there may be significant displacement of the distal fragment posteriorly.

The *anterior humeral line* is a line drawn along the anterior surface of the distal humerus on a true lateral view. Normally this intersects the middle third of the capitellum. If the distal humerus is displaced backwards, it will intersect more anteriorly or not at all (Figures 8.7 and 8.8).

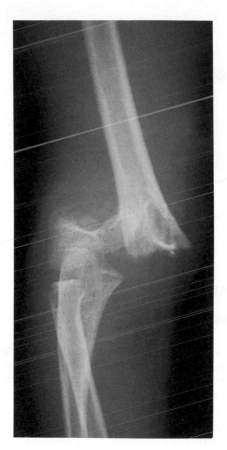

Figure 8.7 A displaced supracondylar fracture.

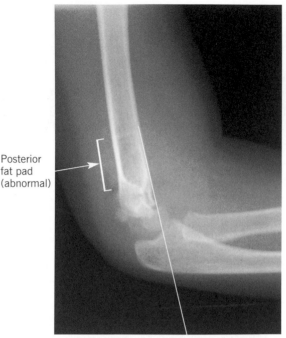

Posterior
fat pad
(abnormal)

Anterior humeral line does not
intersect with middle of capitellum

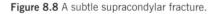

Figure 8.8 A subtle supracondylar fracture.

Management

⚠ **If there is any sign of vascular impairment, call for senior help immediately.**

If there are signs of ischaemia, fracture reduction by gentle traction and extension after appropriate analgesia (see Chapter 3 'Pain Management') will often restore some circulation. All displaced fractures should be referred immediately to orthopaedics. In the absence of displacement or neurovascular signs, treatment of the child is with an above-elbow plaster backslab. Refer to the orthopaedic clinic for follow-up. Despite good management, these fractures are prone to causing a cubitus valgus deformity as the limb grows.

DISLOCATION OF THE ELBOW

For the 'pulled elbow' see the section below (p. 84).

Assessment

Dislocation of the elbow is uncommon in children. On examination the deformity is obvious, with substantial swelling and severe pain. Assess and document the ulnar, median and radial nerve function, and the radial pulse volume and capillary refill.

X-ray

This will typically show a posterolateral dislocation. Associated fractures may occur.

Management

The elbow joint will require reduction, usually under general anaesthesia, as soon as possible. If the circulation is affected, obtain senior help immediately.

MEDIAL EPICONDYLE INJURY

Assessment

This fracture constitutes around 10% of elbow fractures. On examination, there will be tenderness over the prominence of the medial (ulnar side) epicondyle. In particular, test and record ulnar nerve function.

X-ray (Figure 8.9)

There may be minimal or moderate displacement of the medial epicondylar epiphysis. In severe injury, the medial epicondyle may become trapped in the elbow joint. If the child is over 6 years old and the medial epicondylar epiphysis cannot be seen on the anteroposterior view, assume that it has been displaced and lies within the joint. It is easy to mistake the medial epiphysis within the joint for the capitellum.

Management

Refer to orthopaedics if:
- the medial epiphysis is displaced;
- there is evidence of ulnar nerve damage.

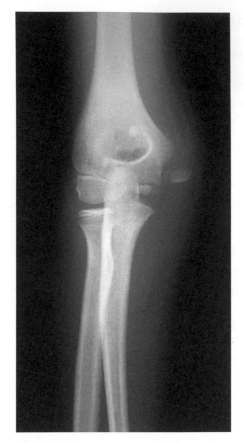

Figure 8.9 A medial epicondylar fracture.

For undisplaced fractures, treatment is with appropriate analgesia, collar and cuff (see Chapter 17 'Practical Procedures') and arrange orthopaedic clinic follow-up.

LATERAL CONDYLE INJURY

Assessment

This constitutes around 20% of elbow fractures. On examination, there will be tenderness on the prominence of the lateral (radial side) condyle.

X-ray

See Figure 8.10.

Management

Refer to orthopaedics for advice.

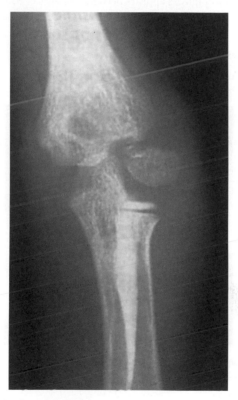

Figure 8.10 A lateral condyle fracture.

OLECRANON FRACTURE

Assessment

These rare fractures are usually due to direct trauma, usually in teenagers. Following a direct blow to the elbow, children are often tender over this area since there is little cushioning; however, if the olecranon is fractured, a large amount of generalized elbow swelling is present.

X-ray

It is easy to confuse the normal epiphysis (Figure 8.11) with a fracture. The normal olecranon epiphysis appears between the ages of 8 and 11, and fuses by the age of 14. Seek senior advice if unsure.

Management

If you see this uncommon injury, seek orthopaedic advice.

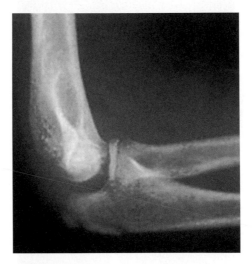

Figure 8.11 A normal olecranon epiphysis.

RADIAL HEAD/NECK FRACTURES

Assessment

The radial head or neck is injured by indirect force, usually a fall on the out-stretched hand. Greenstick fractures of the neck of the radius (Figure 8.12) tend to occur in school-age children, with segmental fractures of the head of the radius (Figure 8.13) in teenagers. On examination, tenderness is hard to

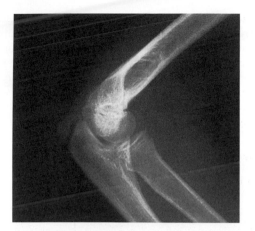

Figure 8.12 Greenstick fracture of the neck of the radius.

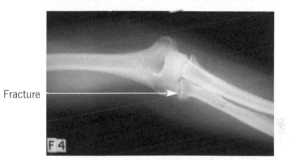

Fracture

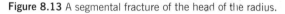

Figure 8.13 A segmental fracture of the head of the radius.

localize but it may be present over the proximal radius, just distal to the lateral epicondyle. There is usually limitation of full extension at the elbow (this may be subtle so compare with the opposite side) and pronation/supination of the forearm is painful.

X-ray

Undisplaced fractures may be extremely difficult to detect on plain X-ray. However, in the presence of clinical signs and a joint effusion, as indicated by a positive fat pad sign (see above), it should be presumed that a fracture is present. In normal patients, the radial head points to the capitellum in all views. Therefore, if the *radiocapitellar line* (a line drawn along the central axis of the radius on the lateral view) does not transect the middle of the capitellum, there is a radial head dislocation and/or a fracture of the radial neck.

Management

Treat the child with a collar and cuff (see Chapter 17 'Practical Procedures') and orthopaedic clinic follow-up.

THE 'PULLED' ELBOW

Assessment

This injury is commonest in children between the ages of one and four following a sudden pull on the arm. Some children are especially prone to the radial head slipping out from the annular ligament, so there may be previous episodes of the same injury. The ligament tightens as the child gets older.

Typical mechanisms would include the hand being grabbed as the child is pulling away, or a jerk while holding hands. As the injury is 'inflicted' by a third party, the history may not be forthcoming or may change. While this should normally ring 'alarm bells' (see Chapter 15 'Non-accidental Injury'), this is guilt driven and, in fact, this injury can occur very easily, without excessive force being applied. Reassurance should be given to those present, since feelings are often running high!

The arm usually lies limp and partially flexed by the child's side. The child will preferentially use the other arm, but may be playing happily. On examination, tenderness may not be elicited. If both the history and the age group are completely classical, no X-ray is required. However, if there is any uncertainty, X-ray to exclude a fracture before attempting manipulation.

Management

Manipulate the elbow (see Chapter 17 'Practical Procedures'), which is a simple procedure that usually gives satisfyingly rapid resolution of symptoms. Review the child after 10 minutes in the playroom. Most will be using the arm happily, and can go home in a collar and cuff, if tolerated (see Chapter 17 'Practical Procedures').

If the child is still not using the arm (which is more common in older toddlers and repeat dislocators), advise the parents that spontaneous reduction will usually take place. If they are still not using the arm in 48 hours, refer for senior advice.

Some children present with repeated dislocations, as it is not always possible to avoid a pull injury (e.g. if the child is trying to run across a road). Parents of repeat dislocators may be happy to be taught the reduction technique.

MIDSHAFT FRACTURES OF THE RADIUS AND/OR ULNA

Usually both bones of the forearm fracture during a fall, or less commonly one bone fractures with a dislocation of the other (see below). With direct trauma, for example, landing on a sharp edge or struck in self-defence, it is possible to fracture a single forearm bone. However, these injuries are relatively uncommon.

Assessment

Fractures of the forearm bones are commonly associated with significant angulation and displacement (Figure 8.14).

Management

For greenstick fractures, up to 30° of angulation will remodel in a toddler. In teenagers, more than 10° is unacceptable. If the angulation is acceptable, place the arm in an above-elbow backslab and refer to an orthopaedic clinic within a day or two. Refer all other fractures for immediate orthopaedic advice.

FRACTURE DISLOCATIONS OF THE FOREARM

There are two patterns of fracture/dislocation: the Monteggia (Figure 8.15), and the Galeazzi (Figure 8.16, p. 88).

A Monteggia injury

This is a rare injury. There is a fracture of the ulna, with associated dislocation of the radial head. This is diagnosed by drawing the radiocapitellar line (see radial head / neck fractures above).

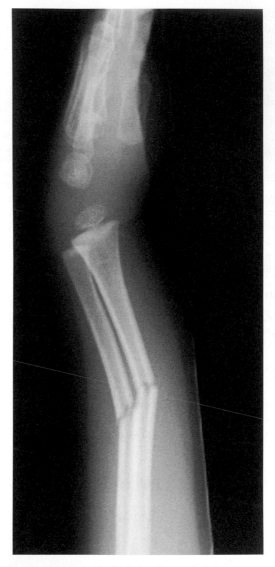

Figure 8.14 Angulated fracture of midshaft radius and ulna.

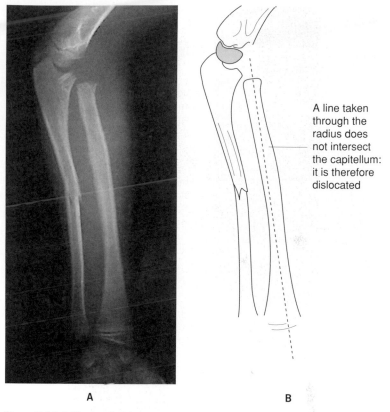

A line taken through the radius does not intersect the capitellum: it is therefore dislocated

A   B

Figure 8.15 A Monteggia injury.

A Galeazzi injury

This occurs in teenagers. There is a fracture of the shaft of radius, associated with a dislocation of the distal ulna.

Management

Refer all fracture dislocations of the radius and ulna for orthopaedic advice.

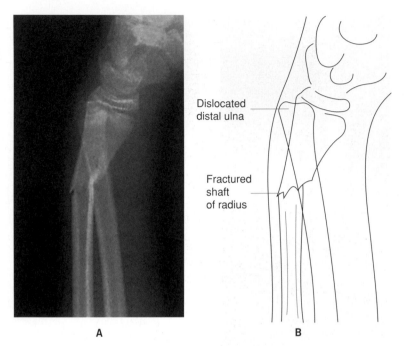

Dislocated
distal ulna

Fractured
shaft
of radius

A   B

Figure 8.16 A Galeazzi injury.

DISTAL RADIUS FRACTURE

Assessment

Fracture of the distal radius is one of the commonest injuries in all age groups, usually occurring after a fall on the outstretched hand. Signs may be subtle. There may be only slight local tenderness, particularly in a young child. At the opposite extreme, there may be obvious deformity, swelling and tenderness over the distal radius.

X-ray

Findings on X-ray vary from a simple undisplaced greenstick or torus fracture (Figure 8.17), or Salter–Harris epiphyseal fracture (see Chapter 7 'Fractures and Dislocations – General'), to severe angulated, displaced fractures of both distal radius and ulna (Figure 8.18).

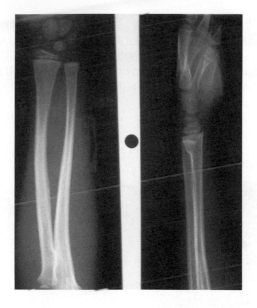

A

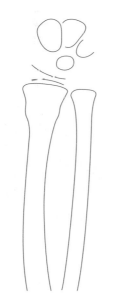

B

Figure 8.17 A torus fracture of the distal radius.

Management

For simple, undisplaced fractures, treat with a forearm plaster of Paris back-slab or splint, and orthopaedic clinic follow-up. Refer to orthopaedics if the fracture is angulated or displaced. Up to 25° of angulation will remodel in a toddler. In teenagers, more than 10° is unacceptable.

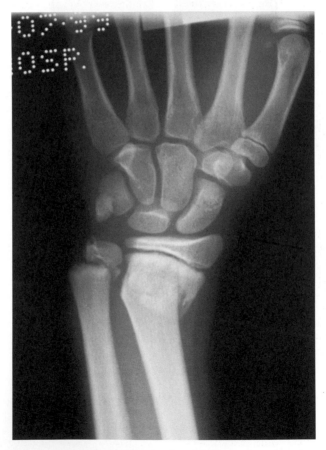

Figure 8.18 Displaced fracture of distal radius and ulna.

SCAPHOID FRACTURE

Scaphoid fractures can only occur once the scaphoid bone has calcified, at around 9 years old. While uncommon, a missed scaphoid fracture may result in very significant disability of the wrist in future years due to non-union or avascular necrosis.

Assessment

Scaphoid injuries are usually caused by a fall on the outstretched hand. There is usually mild swelling on the radial side of the wrist if you look carefully. The signs you should specifically examine for are:
- tenderness in the anatomical snuff box (see Figure 8.19) to gentle pressure (firm pressure will always elicit tenderness in the normal wrist as the superficial branch of the radial nerve traverses this area);
- tenderness over the dorsal aspect of the scaphoid (Figure 8.19);
- tenderness over the palmar aspect of the scaphoid (scaphoid tubercle):
- pain at the wrist when compressing the thumb longitudinally (Figure 8.20);
- pain during passive radial and ulnar deviation of the wrist (Figure 8.21).

X-rays (Figure 8.22)

Ensure you request the appropriate view (see Table 7.1). Four views are usually provided: anteroposterior, lateral, and left and right obliques. Remember that the scaphoid fracture may not be visible on initial films, and arrange review at 10–14 days as further imaging may be necessary (see below).

Management

If you suspect a scaphoid fracture, you must treat the child as if they have one, even if no fracture has been seen on the X-ray films. Place the wrist in a scaphoid plaster cast or a rigid splint with a thumb extension and arrange orthopaedic clinic follow-up (as above).

HAND – GENERAL PRINCIPLES

For general principles see Chapter 9 'Hand Injuries'.

There are some general rules that can be followed for phalangeal and metacarpal fractures, which are listed below.

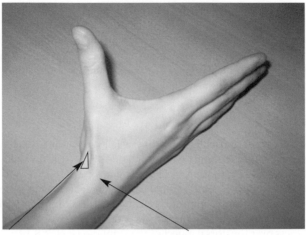

The 'anatomical
snuff box'

Dorsal aspect
of scaphoid

Figure 8.19 The surface anatomy of the scaphoid.

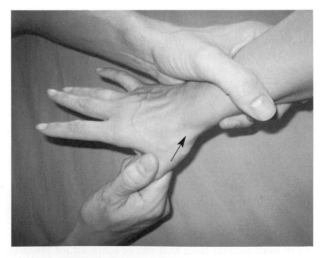

Figure 8.20 'Telescoping' the thumb to elicit pain.

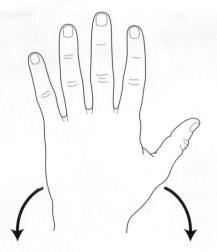

Figure 8.21 Radial and ulnar deviation to elicit pain (pressing on the volar aspect of the scaphoid while you do this will also elicit tenderness).

1 There should be a low threshold for ordering X-rays in hand injuries.
2 Most injuries will cause swelling. Swelling causes stiffness and stiffness causes long-term morbidity, so:

- the hand should be elevated in a high arm sling for a couple of days (see Chapter 17 'Practical Procedures');
- encourage exercises of the fingers;
- if a finger needs support for protection and analgesia, use neighbour strapping (see Chapter 17 'Practical Procedures'). This allows movement in the interphalangeal joints (IPJs).

Examine all hand injuries for finger rotation by making sure that the nails are in a straight line (i.e. parallel) in extension, partial flexion and as the fist closes (see Figure 8.23). The little fingernail may seem rotated but this may be normal: compare with the other side.

Ensure you request the correct X-ray view (see Table 7.1). Note that, if a whole hand view is requested, the views taken are usually an anteroposterior and an oblique view. If a displaced fracture is found, you may require a true lateral view to assess displacement adequately.

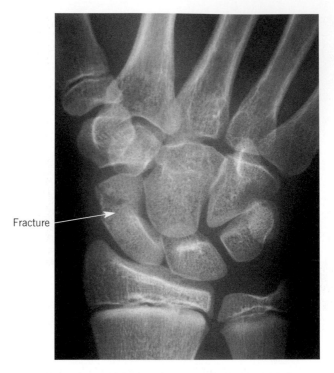

Fracture

Figure 8.22 Fractured scaphoid.

METACARPAL FRACTURES

Assessment

The three main mechanisms are a punch (usually teenagers), a fall on to the hand or, less commonly, a crushing injury. These fractures rarely occur from a glancing blow against an object. Examine carefully for rotational deformity (see above). Both greenstick and epiphyseal injuries may occur.

X-ray (Figure 8.24)

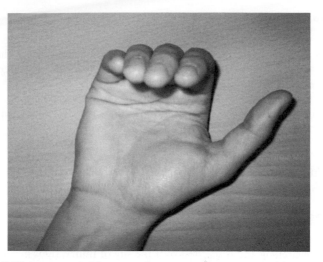

Figure 8.23 Assessment of finger rotation.

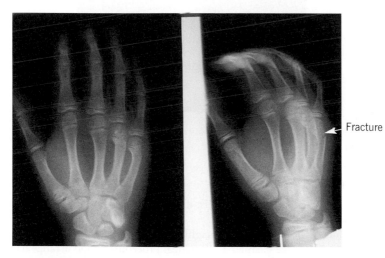

Fracture

Figure 8.24 Fractured neck of the fifth metacarpal - 'boxer's injury'.

Management

Refer to the hand surgery service if there is rotational deformity, angulation greater than 20° in the metaphysis, angulation greater than 45° at the neck of the fifth metacarpal, more than 50% displacement or non-greenstick fractures in three adjacent metacarpals.

For simple metacarpal fractures, apply neighbour strapping to the appropriate digit and elevate the hand in a high arm sling (see Chapter 17 'Practical Procedures'). Arrange hand specialist follow-up.

FRACTURES OF THE PROXIMAL AND MIDDLE PHALANGES

Assessment

These fractures are commonly caused in ball games. Although there may be bruising, swelling and tenderness over the site of injury, signs may be subtle, particularly in the case of little greenstick buckle fractures; therefore, have a low threshold for X-ray.

X-ray (Figure 8.25)

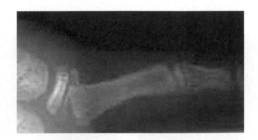

Figure 8.25 Displaced fracture of the base of the proximal phalanx.

Management

Refer to your hand surgery specialist if there is angulation greater than 20° or displacement greater than 50%.

For uncomplicated fractures, neighbour strap the affected digit, place in a high arm sling (see Chapter 17 'Practical Procedures') and arrange hand specialist follow-up.

VOLAR PLATE INJURY

This is an important injury to detect, because it can result in a fixed flexion deformity of the proximal interphalangeal joint (PIPJ). The mechanism is hyperextension, with the child often saying that the finger was 'bent back' (e.g. when catching a large ball or fighting). The complex 'volar plate' of the joint capsule and associated tendons are disrupted and there is usually an associated avulsion fracture.

X-ray

The X-ray findings are subtle and easily missed, unless a true lateral view of the finger is obtained. Even a tiny fragment of bone is a sign of a serious injury (Figure 8.26).

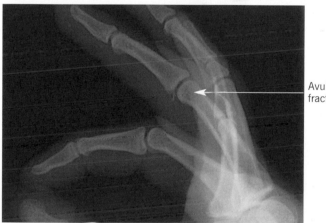

Avulsion
fracture

Figure 8.26 Avulsion fragment of the volar plate at the distal interphalangeal joint.

FRACTURES OF THE DISTAL PHALANX

Fractures of the terminal tuft, neck and base of the distal phalanx are relatively unimportant injuries in themselves. Far more important is any associated fingertip, nailbed or tendon injury (see Chapter 9 'Hand Injuries'). In most cases, all that is required for management of these fractures is elevation in a high arm sling (see Chapter 17 'Practical Procedures') and referral to a hand specialist clinic.

Hand injuries

INTRODUCTION

For fractures of the hand, see Chapter 8 'Injuries of the Upper Limb'.

Hand injuries are common, particularly crush injuries and burns in young children who are exploring their environment, or sports injuries in older children. Most injuries are minor. However, the complexity and density of important structures in the hand make it vulnerable to serious permanent injury. If a significant injury is missed, there may be enormous consequences for a child or young person in terms of loss of function, for their training or occupation.

⚠ **If in doubt about the extent of a hand injury, always seek expert advice.**

Consult your local policy for referral procedures, since hand specialists may be part of the orthopaedic, plastic surgery or emergency department services, and referral may depend on the nature of the injury.

Hand injuries frequently swell. Swelling causes pain and stiffness. This may be prevented by elevation to shoulder level in a 'high arm sling' (see Chapter 17 'Practical Procedures'), if the child will cooperate. This helps to alleviate pain, and is necessary for a day or two if swelling is present or likely.

⚠ **Rings should always be removed at triage to prevent swelling and ischaemia of a digit.**

⚠ Use X-rays: *essential* for wounds caused by glass; *advisable* for any injury if fracture possible.

Refer to Chapter 17 'Practical Procedures' for the following procedures: a digital nerve block for analgesia; a high arm sling; neighbour strapping; and how to trephine a nail.

CLINICAL EXAMINATION

A methodical, slick system for examining hands is essential, albeit with modifications for young children. To do this, an understanding of the underlying anatomy is needed. Sometimes exploration under general anaesthetic is required for thorough examination or to exclude injury.

The infant or pre-school child

Small children are unable to obey the simple commands needed to test hand function. You are, therefore, dependent on observation of function, posture and some limited tests. Look for the 'cascade' of normal finger posture (Figure 9.1),which is disrupted when flexor tendons are severed.

Fortunately in this age group, most structures are flexible so that fractures are less likely, and unless there is a laceration, tendons, ligaments and nerves are generally intact. Secondly, the longer-term complications of stiffness and disability are less likely, since young children will continue to use their hands despite injury.

Older children

Firstly, *ask*:
• which hand do you use to write with?
• (if laceration is present) does your hand or your fingers feel funny or numb anywhere?

Look for:
• deformity;
• swelling;
• distribution of lacerations.

Test for:
• range of movement of affected joints;
• function of individual tendons;

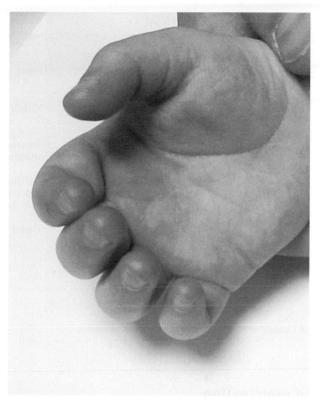

Figure 9.1 Normal finger cascade.

- function of specific nerves;
- sensation.

⚠️ **Draw diagrams.**

It is much easier to interpret written notes if diagrams are used. Most emergency departments have ink pads and stamps.

Use the right terminology when writing notes:
- avoid 'medial' and 'lateral', but rather describe as 'radial' and 'ulnar';
- do not number fingers (second, third, etc).

The abbreviations shown in Figures 9.2 and 9.3 are well known and generally acceptable.

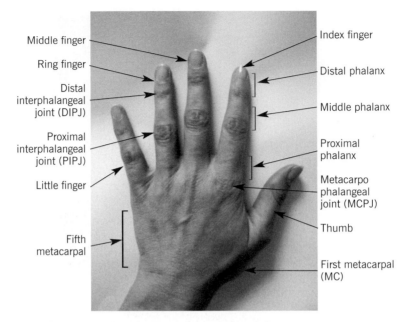

Middle finger
Ring finger
Distal interphalangeal joint (DIPJ)
Proximal interphalangeal joint (PIPJ)
Little finger
Fifth metacarpal

Index finger
Distal phalanx
Middle phalanx
Proximal phalanx
Metacarpo phalangeal joint (MCPJ)
Thumb
First metacarpal (MC)

Figure 9.2 Dorsum of hand – description and abbreviations.

Tendon examination

Extensor tendons

Ask the child to bring their fingers out straight, and not to let you bend them as you test strength against resistance. Make this into a game, competing for strength. Observe any inability to extend fully. Remember that swelling or pain may sometimes prevent full extension. A finger with a partially severed tendon may look fully extended, but there will be weakness and pain when resisting flexion.

Flexor tendons

You need to understand the relationship of the two layers of tendons in order to understand the examination (see Figure 9.4).

To test the *superficial tendons*, evaluate each individual finger in turn. Ask the child to place the hand, palm side up, on a flat surface. Then ask them to bend each finger, in turn, as you hold all the others down. The finger should flex at the MCPJ and PIPJ.

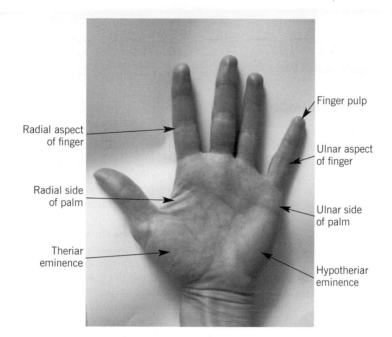

Figure 9.3 Volar or palmar aspect of the hand – descriptions.

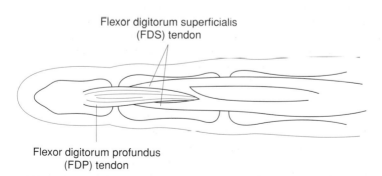

Figure 9.4 Relationship of the flexor tendons.

To test the *profundus tendons*, again evaluate each individual finger in turn. Immobilize each finger against the flat surface, palm side up, by pressing down on the middle phalanx. Ask the child to bend the tip of the finger. The finger should flex at the DIPJ.

Nerve examination

Sensory function

Test for sensation by asking if light touch feels *normal*. Do not ask the child simply if they can feel it, as sensation is rarely completely absent, and proprioception and some feeling will be present owing to other factors. Ask if it feels the same as uninjured areas, because 'not quite normal' in localized areas often implies nerve damage. Use words such as 'strong' or 'fuzzy' so children can understand the concept.

The distribution of the sensory territories of the three major nerves may be quite variable. Damage to these large trunks occurs proximal to the wrist, so is unusual. The most reliable places to test are the first web space for the radial nerve, the index fingertip for the median nerve and the little fingertip for the ulnar nerve(Figures 9.5 and 9.6). Far more commonly, the digital nerves are damaged. There are two main trunks for each digit, which run along the ulnar and radial sides dorsally, with equivalent palmar branches (see Figure 9.7). Again, absence of sensation is relative, not absolute.

Motor function

Always compare with the opposite hand, as loss of power is rarely absolute.
- The *radial nerve* supplies the wrist and finger extensors, which should be able to strongly resist flexion.
- The *median nerve* is best assessed by testing opposition. Ask the child to touch the tip of the thumb to the tip of the little finger, and to stop you 'breaking the ring'.
- The *ulnar nerve* innervates most of the intrinsic muscles of the hand. A simple test is to put your pen between child's little and ring fingers, and ask them to stop you pulling it out.

Wound exploration

Having reassured yourself that there is no damage to underlying structures by clinical examination, you should always confirm this by exploring any deep wound under local anaesthetic. Anything that glistens or looks white may be a tendon. Examine through the full range of movement, as severed tendons may retract and hide.

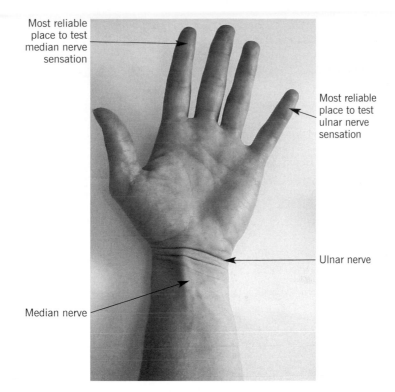

Most reliable place to test median nerve sensation

Most reliable place to test ulnar nerve sensation

Ulnar nerve

Median nerve

Figure 9.5 Path and distribution of the median and ulnar nerves.

⚠ Do not extend a wound in order to explore it.

Sometimes it can be difficult to assess a wound because of bleeding and a tourniquet is required to create a bloodless field. In such cases, referral to a specialist is advised.

⚠ Seek advice if ever in doubt when exploring a wound.

FINGERTIP INJURIES

Fingertips are complex anatomical structures that are frequently injured (most often shut in doors). These crush injuries are very stressful to

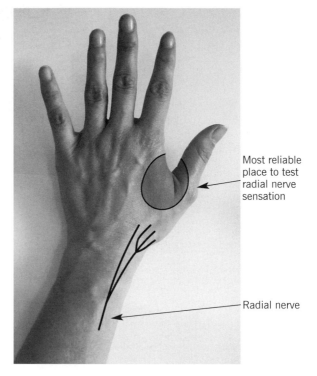

Most reliable place to test radial nerve sensation

Radial nerve

Figure 9.6 Path and distribution of the radial nerve.

children and their families. Consider intranasal diamorphine or oral morphine, for both pain and anxiety (see Chapter 3 'Pain Management'). Confusingly, these injuries evoke widely differing opinions in their management. Unfortunately, robust, long-term outcome studies do not exist to assist you in your decisions.

General principles

The main principles of management are as follows.
- Children's fingertips are extremely good at regenerating themselves, thus conservative management is possible in most cases. This is particularly true for toenail injuries.

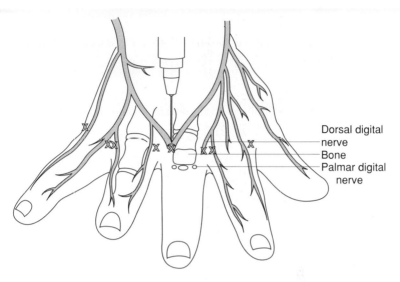

Figure 9.7 Distribution of the digital nerves.

- Restoration of normal anatomy is the aim. Much can be achieved with adhesive strips, tissue glue and dressings. Sutures are not usually needed.
- Long-term problems may occur at the base of the nail if the skin of the nailfold is allowed to adhere on to the germinal matrix, resulting in abnormal growth of the new nail into the nailbed. This must be prevented (see below).
- Try to determine the presence or absence of a *nailbed laceration*. In many cases this is an educated guess. A practical approach needs to be taken because of the lack of evidence base for the necessity of repair and the fact that this procedure in children often requires a general anaesthetic in an operating theatre, with a hand surgeon. The presence of a subungual haematoma larger than 50% of the nail or an underlying fracture make a nailbed laceration more likely.
- Always use non-adherent dressings, e.g. paraffin-impregnated gauze (such as Jelonet®) or a silicon-based dressing (such as Mepitel®).

History

Ask about the timing and mechanism of injury, e.g. doors, windows and hand dominance.

Examination

It helps to think methodically about the different components of the finger-tip. Assess for:

- haemostasis;
- bone exposure;
- skin contusion and viability;
- contamination;
- avulsion of the nail from the germinal matrix under cuticle;
- anatomical stability;
- subungual haematoma.

Management

This depends on findings on examination (above). Since the exact injuries are highly variable, the principles outlined below will guide you.

⚠ Most crush injuries require an X-ray.

Bleeding profusely

Elevate in a high arm sling (see Chapter 17 'Practical Procedures') for 10 minutes with a compression, non-adhesive dressing and bandage until further assessment possible.

Bone exposure or skin jeopardized

If bone is exposed, or the skin is very contused, contaminated or non-viable, refer to a specialist. For injuries proximal to the DIPJ, every attempt should be made to preserve the amputated part. It should be covered with sterile, soaked dressings, sealed in a plastic bag and placed on ice. The remaining finger should be covered with a non-adherent dressing, and elevated in a high arm sling.

Skin or pulp missing

This will grow back quickly. An area less than the size of the child's nail will require non-adhesive dressings (e.g. Mepitel® or Jelonet®) for a week or so. Larger areas should be referred to a specialist clinic.

Nail and nailbed injuries (Figure 9.8)

Nails grow from the base. The gap in the nailfold must not be allowed to close or normal longitudinal growth of the new nail may not occur. Similarly, a large nailbed laceration will affect the growth of the new nail. Not only will the defect be cosmetic, but it may be painful.

If the nail is very loose, remove the nail and inspect the nailbed. If the nail is quite firmly adherent, attempts should not be made to remove it as this causes further damage. Seek advice. Deep lacerations are likely to involve the nailbed but, if distal, can be managed conservatively.

If the nail has already been avulsed or you have had to remove it, it must be replaced back in the nailfold (Figure 9.9). Various techniques can be employed. First clean the nail and trim any attached skin. If the nail is lost, a substitute splint must be inserted. This may be custom made using the wax paper backing of Jelonet® dressings. Once in position, a combination of tissue glue across the nailfold with adhesive strips over the fingertip is usually sufficient to keep it in place for a week or two.

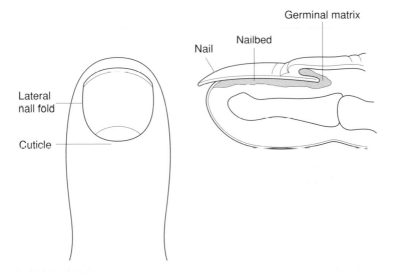

Figure 9.8 The nail and nailbed.

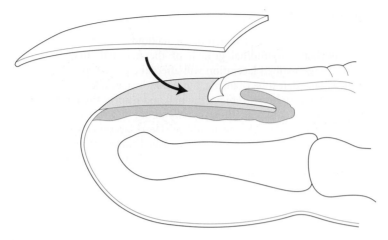

Figure 9.9 Nail being reinserted into the nailfold.

Anatomically unstable injuries

Large burst-type lacerations (Figure 9.10) or those involving more than 50% of the digital circumference are likely to be anatomically unstable and require sutures. Milder lacerations can usually be maintained with adhesive strips and a supportive dressing.

If suturing through nail is required, this can be quite difficult. If the nail is avulsed, one suture each side can be taken first through the skin, then through the nail separately. Each can then be pulled tight, bringing the nail into position, as a second stage.

Subungual haematoma

Crush injuries to fingertips may cause a subungual haematoma. This is a collection of blood underneath the nail because the nailbed has torn but the overlying nail has remained intact. The blood under the nail may escape out of the side of the nail, but often becomes trapped underneath, causing pressure to build up in this very sensitive area. Trephining the nail releases the blood and is a very satisfying procedure because of the instant relief of symptoms. (see Chapter 17 'Practical Procedures').

A haematoma larger than 50% of the nail makes a nailbed laceration likely (see above).

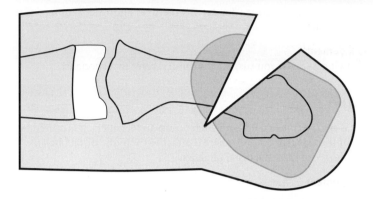

Figure 9.10 A burst-type laceration..

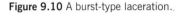

Underlying fracture

For all except minor injuries, an X-ray should be performed. If a fracture is present, but confined to the shaft of the distal phalanx and undisplaced, a simple dressing may be applied and oral flucloxacillin prescribed if the skin is broken. If the fracture is through the epiphyseal plate, refer to a specialist.

TENDON AND LIGAMENT INJURIES

See above for assessment. All suspected injuries should be referred immediately to a specialist.

Ulnar collateral ligament injury

This is a rare injury, and usually occurs in older children. A forced abduction of the thumb, for example, from ski poles, results in instability of the ulnar collateral ligament, which runs from the thumb metacarpal to the base of the proximal phalanx, on the ulnar side. It does not usually tear, but is associated with an avulsion-type fracture,

Salter–Harris type 2 (see Chapter 7 'Fractures and Dislocations – General Approach').

Management
Following X-ray, if you suspect this injury, refer to a specialist.

Mallet finger

This is also an unusual injury, which occurs in teenagers. It is caused by rupture of the extensor tendon where it attaches on to the distal phalanx. There is obvious droop of the distal phalanx.

Management
X-ray to see if there is an associated fracture. Immobilize with the digit in slight hyperextension and refer to your hand service as an outpatient. Explain to the patient that this will take around 6 weeks to heal. During this time the splint must be worn at all times. It needs to be removed to wash the digit, but flexion must be absolutely prevented during these times. For hygiene, and to avoid macerated skin, a Zimmer splint™ (aluminium with foam backing) can be custom made to cover the dorsum of the digit, curving round to incorporate the DIPJ. This is better than the traditional plastic mallet splint.

Volar plate injury

See Chapter 8 'Injuries of the Upper Limb', pp. 96–7.

Nerve injuries

See above for assessment.

Management
All suspected injuries should be referred immediately to a specialist, with the exception of loss of sensation of a digital nerve, distal to the DIPJ.

INFECTIONS

Paronychia

This is a localized infection, usually around the cuticle. It is commonly caused by biting the nails. Once the infection has progressed from the reddened stage to develop a collection of pus, antibiotics are useless; drainage is required.

Management

Incision and drainage is required. A digital block may be needed (see Chapter 17 'Practical Procedures'). If a large collection of pus is visible, this may not be necessary as the overlying skin is dead. Insert a scalpel blade directly into the pus, then 'milk' the finger to extrude all pus. Cover with a non-adherent dressing and advise the patient to soak their finger in warm water twice over the next 24 hours, milking any remaining pus out.

If a paronychia is recurrent, consider the presence of underlying osteomyelitis and request an X-ray.

Tendon infection

Any wound infection may cause tendon infection. Flexor tendons are contained within synovial sheaths, and infection can spread rapidly and be extremely destructive. This is heralded by pain, erythema, swelling and pain on passive extension.

⚠ Refer immediately to a hand specialist, if you have any suspicion of flexor tendon infection.

Pulp and palmar space infections

A collection of pus in the pulp space is called a felon. The finger pulp is hot, red, swollen, fluctuant and extremely painful. Refer to a hand specialist.

The palm contains soft tissue spaces, confined by fascial compartments. If infection occurs, signs may be subtle because it is deep seated. Look for the loss of the normal dip between the metacarpals and test for pain on compression.

⚠ Refer immediately to a hand specialist if you have any suspicion of a palmar space infection.

CUT WRISTS IN DELIBERATE SELF-HARM

This is unusual under the age of 16, but you must be aware of it because of the very serious nature of this behaviour starting at such a young age. The child may not be forthcoming about the mechanism and may invent another history.

⚠ **Suspect deliberate self-harm if you ever see superficial lacerations on the insides of the wrists.**

Deliberate self-harm must be taken seriously, and a full psychosocial assessment performed by an experienced multidisciplinary team.

REFLEX SYMPATHETIC DYSTROPHY

This is a dysautonomia, which occurs from the age of 8 or so. It may or may not follow injury, but can present quite dramatically with pallor, coldness, hyperaesthesia, swelling or stiffness of a limb, commonly the forearm and hand. Milder autonomic nervous system symptoms occur temporarily quite frequently in teenage girls with hand or ankle injuries, and can be mistaken for fractures or dislocations with vascular injury. There may be a very abnormal posture but the overriding feature is severe pain.

Delay in diagnosis is common and frequently follows multiple radiological imaging and prolonged immobilization, which usually make things worse.

Management

Reassure the patient and parent that there is no severe injury. Do not immobilize the affected part. Do not discharge without arranging follow-up by someone experienced with these problems. The condition responds to physiotherapy, often with psychological input.

10

Injuries of the lower limb

SLIPPED UPPER FEMORAL EPIPHYSIS

This condition occurs in children around puberty, before the femoral epiphysis has fused, between 8 and 15 years. It is more common in boys and the aetiology is thought to be partly hormonal. Two body types are classically, though not necessarily, associated with this condition:

• obesity with underdeveloped genitalia; and
• tall and thin with normal sexual development.

The actual slipping of the femoral epiphysis may occur gradually or suddenly, and may or may not follow trauma (which may be minor). The condition may be bilateral.

⚠ There may or may not be a history of trauma.

Minor trauma can precipitate a slipped femoral epiphysis, but many parents try to associate limping with recent trauma, which is often a 'red herring'.

Assessment

The child may be limping or non-weight-bearing. On examination hip movements, particularly rotation, may be limited by pain.

X-ray

X-ray the whole pelvis to help you to compare with the opposite side, but beware of bilateral disease. Subtle slips are better seen on a true lateral. However, to reduce the amount of radiation, a compromise is a 'frog leg' lateral view, where the legs are partly externally rotated. A line drawn along the superior border of the femoral neck should normally cut through the top of the epiphysis. In a slipped upper femoral epiphysis (Figure 10.1), the whole of the epiphysis may lie below this line (see below). If in doubt, seek senior

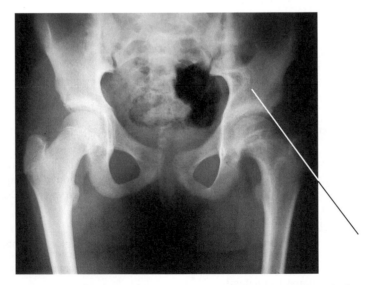

Figure 10.1 Left slipped upper femoral epiphysis. 'A line drawn through the trochanteric epiphysis and along the neck of the femur should partly bisect the head. Note here the head is completely below the line. Compare this with the opposite side'.

advice. Further imaging, such as a radioisotope bone scan, may be needed for diagnosis.

Management

If you suspect a slipped upper femoral epiphysis, seek orthopaedic advice.

PERTHES' AVASCULAR NECROSIS OF THE FEMORAL HEAD

This is caused by avascular necrosis of the femoral head. It usually affects children in the 6–11 age group. Anything that affects the vasculature of the small vessels that supply the femoral head, via the capsule and the *ligamentum teres*, can cause Perthes' disease. This includes haematological conditions, abnormal anatomy or steroid treatment. The condition may be bilateral.

⚠ There may or may not be a history of trauma.

Minor trauma can precipitate Perthes' disease, but many parents try to associate limping with recent trauma, which is often a 'red herring'.

Assessment

The child may be limping or non-weight-bearing. On examination, hip movements, particularly rotation, may be limited by pain.

X-ray (Figure 10.2)

X-ray the whole pelvis to help you to compare with the opposite side but beware of bilateral disease. In the initial stages, subtle osteomalacia is seen of the femoral head. Later, it becomes flattened, with a 'moth-eaten' appearance, patchy sclerosis and widening of the joint space. If in doubt, seek senior advice. Further imaging, such as magnetic resonance imaging, may be needed for diagnosis.

Management

If you suspect Perthes' disease, seek orthopaedic advice.

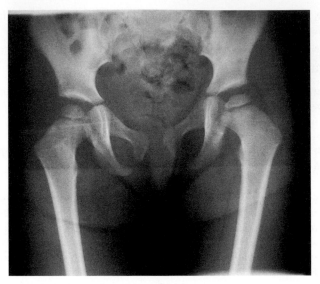

A

Increased joint space compared with the right hip

Femoral head smaller and flatter than the right

B

Figure 10.2 Left Perthes' disease.

TRANSIENT SYNOVITIS OR IRRITABLE HIP

An 'irritable hip' is a diagnosis of exclusion. In particular, septic arthritis, slipped upper femoral epiphysis, Perthes' disease and juvenile chronic arthritis should be considered. The most common age group is toddlers and early school-age children. The aetiology is unsure but it may be a reaction to a viral illness.

Signs may be mild (intermittent, slight limp) or more severe (non-weight-bearing and marked decrease in range of movement).

Management

This depends on your local policy, and depends on the severity of symptoms and risk of other pathology. Investigations may include X-ray, ultrasound, white cell count, C-reactive protein and erythrocyte sedimentation rate. All these investigations are performed to screen for other diseases, except for ultrasound, where needle aspiration may provide symptomatic relief.

Transient synovitis is a benign condition and does not usually recur. Since it is a diagnosis of exclusion, all cases should be followed up in an appropriate clinic to ensure return to normal within 2 weeks and lack of development of any new symptoms.

AVULSION FRACTURES AROUND THE HIP

Children may sustain avulsion fractures following sudden movements, usually during sport. Examples include the ischial tuberosity, and the greater and lesser trochanters of the femur. The clue is in the history. The child may or may not be able to bear weight. X-ray if in doubt, although most are managed conservatively unless significant displacement is present.

FEMORAL SHAFT FRACTURES

Assessment

Considerable force is required to fracture the femur.

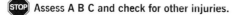 Assess A B C and check for other injuries.

Femoral shaft fractures alone can be responsible for significant bleeding, although in isolation will not cause clinical signs of shock.

Assessment

Diagnosis is usually obvious. There is often significant swelling of the affected thigh, with associated tenderness. The child will be unable to bear weight or lift the limb off the bed. In infants and toddlers with chubby thighs, signs are more subtle. Assess and record distal neurovascular status.

 In infants or toddlers check the history (see Chapter 15 'Non-accidental Injury').

Fractures may be transverse, spiral or supracondylar.

⚠ **A spiral fracture of the femur is highly suspicious of non-accidental injury.**

Management

The child will require opiate analgesia and ideally a femoral nerve block before splintage, then moving to X-ray (see Chapter 3 'Pain Management', and Chapter 17 'Practical Procedures').

Following radiographic confirmation, refer to an orthopaedic surgeon. All will be admitted in the first instance. Younger children will be placed in traction (Gallows' for infants, skin traction for older children), and children over 5 years may be considered for internal fixation.

INJURIES OF THE KNEE

Most are sprains, sustained during sport or twisting while falling over. Major fractures of the knee are very uncommon in children, unless severe trauma has been sustained. Osteochondral fractures may result in fragments within the joint itself.

Assessment

Accurate assessment can be difficult acutely because of pain. Assess whether the child is bearing weight, for the presence of an effusion, the range of movement, the ability to extend fully and whether the ligaments are intact.

Ligamentous injury
Children are stretchy. Therefore, serious ligamentous injury is unusual. When assessing for injury, assess the normal side first to see how stretchy it is and to gain the child's confidence.

To assess the collateral ligaments, place your knee underneath the child's so it can relax, partially flexed. Palpate for focal tenderness. The medial collateral runs from the medial femoral condyle to the medial aspect of the tibia. The lateral collateral runs from the lateral femoral condyle to the fibula. Then gently stress the ligaments by encouraging relaxation, resting one hand on the thigh, taking the lower leg and exerting valgus and varus distraction.

To assess the cruciate ligaments, again let the patient's knee rest on your thigh. Grasp the upper calf with both hands, and push and pull to look for instability.

Meniscal injury

This is best assessed with the child lying prone. Flex the knee and, while gently pushing the heel so the knee is into the bed, rotate the foot clockwise and anticlockwise. The rotation causes pain, if meniscal injury is present.

Indications for X-ray

X-ray if completely non-weight-bearing, if there is a large effusion or if the mechanism is significant.

Indications for same-day orthopaedic referral

Inability to extend fully is called a 'locked knee'. If this is present (despite coaxing!) refer. Seek advice for all fractures. Other injuries can be reviewed in an orthopaedic clinic. Apply a compression bandage or splint (detachable 'cricket' splints are very useful) and issue crutches. Advise 'RICE' (see the section on sprains in Chapter 4 'Wounds and Soft Tissue Injuries').

PATELLAR FRACTURE

Assessment

Fractures of the patella caused by a direct trauma are rare in childhood. More commonly a 'sleeve' fracture occurs on sudden quadriceps contraction, such as while jumping. The inferior pole of the patella is avulsed. There will be pain and swelling around the patella, and difficulty extending the knee or performing a straight leg raise.

X-ray

X-rays may not be diagnostic. Do not mistake the congenital bipartite patella for a fracture. This accessory bone is found in the upper, outer quadrant of the patella on the anteroposterior view and the edges are rounded.

Management

Refer for orthopaedic advice if you suspect this injury.

PATELLAR DISLOCATION

Assessment

This often follows a direct blow to the medial side of the knee but may happen spontaneously. It is most frequently seen in adolescent girls. On examination, the patient usually holds the knee in flexion, and there is obvious lateral displacement of the patella.

Management

Reduction of a dislocated patella can often be achieved using Entonox for its analgesic and sedative effect. Ensure the child is able to use the breath-activated mechanism. Entonox should be inhaled for 2–3 minutes prior to attempting reduction of the dislocation. Once the child is more comfortable, reduce the patella by firm pressure over the lateral aspect, with both thumbs, while an assistant gently extends the leg. After the patella is reduced, apply a full-length cylinder plaster or splint ('cricket' splint) and arrange orthopaedic clinic follow-up.

OSGOOD–SCHLATTER'S DISEASE

Assessment

This is thought to be a traction apophysitis of the patellar tendon as it inserts into the proximal tibia, particularly common in sporty children. It occurs in late childhood and early adolescence, and is more common in boys.

A lump is seen or felt around the tibial tuberosity, which may be tender.

X-ray

X-rays are not necessary if the clinical picture is characteristic.

Management

The child should be advised to reduce their level of activity according to the pain. This is a difficult trade-off and some will continue normal sports. This is not harmful. The condition is self-limiting over a year or two.

FRACTURES OF THE TIBIA AND FIBULA

Assessment

Isolated fractures of either the tibia or fibula require significant trauma, either direct or by twisting. Greenstick-type fractures occur.

The commonest fracture is seen in very young children, from learning to walk until approximately 4 years old. Minor twisting trauma may result in an oblique, undisplaced fracture, otherwise known as a 'toddler's fracture'. It may even occur on standing up suddenly.

On examination, there may be little to find, except a limping child. There is no swelling and direct pressure often does not elicit tenderness. The clue is in twisting the foot, to cause torsion of tibia, which elicits pain.

X-ray

The diagnosis may be obvious, but subtle greenstick fractures and toddler's fractures, can be difficult to diagnose. In a toddler's fracture (Figure 10.3), the periosteum can hold the bone so tightly that displacement does not occur, and there may be no apparent X-ray changes. However, around 10 days later, reabsorption along the fracture line and callus at the outer cortex are visible. Unlike other spiral fractures, toddler's fractures are not suspicious of non-accidental injury.

⚠ **If you suspect a toddler's fracture and the X-ray is normal, immobilize the leg in a plaster and re-X-ray after 10 days.**

Management

Undisplaced greenstick fractures and toddler's fractures may be immobilized in an above-knee plaster cast. For all other fractures, obtain an orthopaedic opinion: surgery may be required, or at least elevation and observation as an in-patient because of the risk of compartment syndrome.

ANKLE INJURIES

Assessment

Ankle fractures are uncommon in childhood and, if present, tend to be greenstick or Salter–Harris epiphyseal type fractures. The child may be able

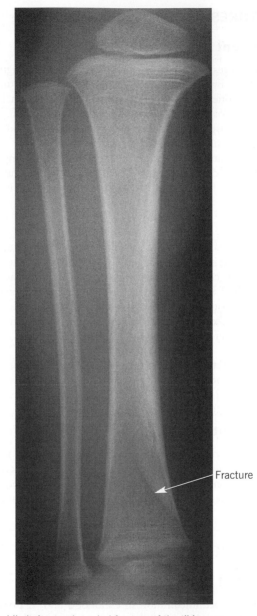

Fracture

Figure 10.3 A 'toddler's fracture' – spiral fracture of the tibia.

to partially weight-bear, despite the presence of a fracture. Similarly, the ligaments either side of the joint are not usually significantly unstable.

Children may present quite dramatically with severe pain, an altered posture and a cold foot, which is a temporary phenomenon and shares features with reflex sympathetic dystrophy (see Chapter 9 'Hand Injuries').

Is it just a sprain? The 'Ottawa ankle rules'

These well-known rules for imaging in adult injuries probably apply to older children but have not been validated in children younger than 8 years. For teenagers, no radiological imaging is needed, if the tenderness is localized to the anterior part of either malleolus, or if they can bear weight for more than two steps (either at the time of the injury or while being examined).

X-rays

It is important to check that the joint is stable, by checking that the gap between the talus and the tibia and fibula is parallel (Figure 10.4). Look for small avulsion fractures of the lateral malleolus.

Management

Fractures

Refer immediately if there is any talar shift or a displaced fracture. For simple, undisplaced fractures, apply a below-knee plaster cast. Small avulsion fractures can be treated as a sprain. Arrange orthopaedic clinic follow-up.

Sprains

There is little evidence of benefit from bandaging, although a compression bandage such as Tubigrip™ may help reduce swelling. In the first 24 hours, ice packs can help reduce swelling. Significant swelling is unusual but, if present, 24 hours' rest and elevation above hip level is recommended.

Children recover from sprains quickly and the use of crutches should be discouraged, if partially weight-bearing. Teenagers may take up to 3 weeks to recover and should be followed up in an appropriate clinic to encourage a normal gait.

Proprioception can be affected long term, unless balancing exercises are practised. Ask the child to stand on one leg and they will see how 'wobbly' the affected side is compared with the other leg. They should practise balancing on one foot several times a day, for example, when brushing teeth or standing on the bed before getting in.

If the child is sporty, referral for physiotherapy is beneficial, so that he or she may return to normal activities as soon as possible.

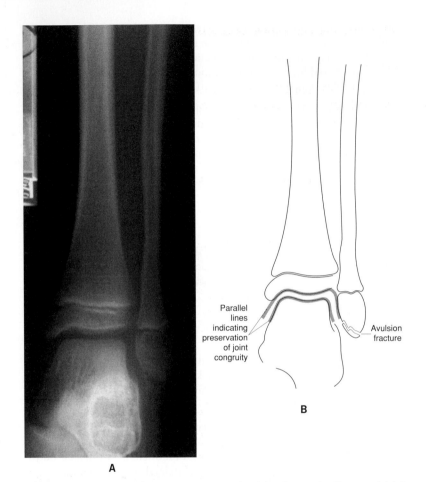

Parallel
lines
indicating
preservation
of joint
congruity

Avulsion
fracture

B

A

Figure 10.4 Fracture of the lateral malleolus (avulsion fracture) with normal joint congruity.

CALCANEUM FRACTURE

Assessment

The commonest cause of a calcaneal fracture is a fall from a height, landing on the heels, from mid-childhood onwards. There is swelling and weight-bearing is very painful.

⚠ Always assess the spine for associated injury.

X-ray

It is important to request calcaneal views specifically, as normal anteroposterior and lateral views of the foot may not reveal a calcaneal fracture. Do not confuse the calcaneal epiphysis with a fracture.

Management

Refer in case further imaging (computed tomography) or admission for analgesia and elevation is needed.

FRACTURE OF THE PROXIMAL FIFTH METATARSAL

Assessment

These are usually caused by an inversion injury, causing *peroneus brevis* to avulse its bony attachment. On examination there is usually localized tenderness.

X-ray

Do not mistake the epiphysis (Figure 10.5), which lies parallel to the shaft of the fifth metatarsal, for a fracture (Figure 10.6). However, the epiphysis itself may be avulsed or fractured.

Management

For undisplaced fractures, either a below-knee plaster cast or simply crutches, depending on the child's ability to bear weight and on patient preference. Arrange orthopaedic clinic follow-up.

OTHER METATARSAL INJURIES

Greenstick fractures of one or more metatarsals occur in small children when jumping from a height, e.g. bed. Older children may sustain greenstick, epiphyseal or transverse fractures. Stress fractures may occur in athletic children. For multiple or displaced fractures, apply a below-knee

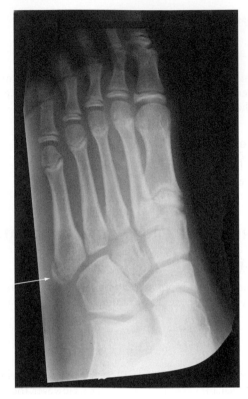

Figure 10.5 Normal epiphysis of the fifth metatarsal.

plaster cast. Otherwise, simply rest and elevation for a day or two is all that is required. Arrange orthopaedic clinic follow-up.

TOE INJURIES

Stubbed and crushed toes are common. Dislocations are unusual but can be reduced under a digital block (see Chapter 17 'Practical Procedures'). Treatment of nail and distal injuries is similar to fingertip injuries (see Chapter 9 'Hand Injuries'), although usually less aggressive. Management of fractures is difficult and consists of common-sense measures, such as

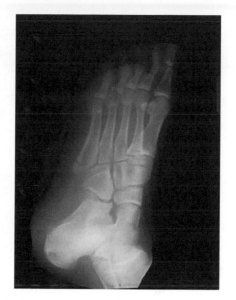

Figure 10.6 Fractured base of the fifth metatarsal.

elevation, crutches and wide-fitting shoes. For this reason, X-rays are unnecessary unless involvement of the metatarsal is suspected. Neighbour strapping may be of benefit after the initial swelling subsides.

11

Burns, scalds, and chemical and electrical injuries

INTRODUCTION

Burn injury is the second commonest cause of accidental death in children in the UK. Children in social class 5 are 15 times more likely to die in a house fire than those in social class 1. Many of these deaths are due to inhalation injury with only minor skin burns.

 Minor burns with inhalational injury can kill. Obtain senior advice if it is possible that smoke or fumes have been inhaled.

Most minor burn injuries occur in the home in children under the age of 3 years, and are due to hot liquids or are contact burns. They are not life threatening, but they may leave permanent scars or abnormalities in pigmentation of the skin. Many such injuries are preventable, for example, kettles and hot drinks should not be in easy reach and hot irons should not be left on the floor. Sunburn can occur, owing to lack of protection in hot weather or during the misuse of sunbeds.

DEFINITIONS

A *burn* is the response of the skin and subcutaneous tissues to thermal energy generated by heat, chemicals, electricity, radiation, etc. A *scald* is a burn produced by a hot liquid and vapour.

CAUSES

Burn injury may be caused by:
- liquid spillage;
- contact;
- fire/flame/flash;
- radiation, including sunburn;
- friction;
- electricity;
- chemicals.

HISTORY

A careful history must be taken of every detail of the incident that led to the burn injury, particularly the time of events and the action taken by parents. Your history needs to take the following factors into account.
- The risk of inhalational injury: possible exposure to smoke or hot gases in a house fire.
- The risk of associated injuries, for example, injuries sustained while trying to escape a fire.
- The likely depth of the burn. This depends on the temperature and the duration of contact. Burns from hot fat or oil, and those from exhaust pipes may be full thickness.
- The patient at risk of having a deeper burn owing to a sensory impairment, for example in cerebral palsy or during an epileptic fit.
- A delay in presentation, which may imply non-accidental injury (see Chapter 15).

(STOP) **If any of the above 'alarm bells' are present, seek senior advice.**

Remember to check the tetanus immunization state of the child (see Chapter 4 'Wounds and Soft Tissue Injuries').

EXAMINATION

All patients with burn injury must have an assessment of:
- Airway (with cervical spine control if appropriate);
- Breathing;
- Circulation.

See Figure 11.1.

(STOP) **If a patient needs resuscitation, this is a major burn. Go back to A, B, C and seek senior advice. Refer to APLS guidelines.**

Assessment of airway and breathing

The more detailed management of inhalational injury is outside the remit of this book.

⚠ **Do not forget to check for carbon monoxide poisoning, if there was a fire within an enclosed space.**

Remember that carboxyhaemoglobin levels do not always correlate with severity of carbon monoxide poisoning. If carboxyhaemoglobin levels are above 3% or you are worried about symptoms, such as headache or mild confusion, seek advice from your local poisons unit (in the UK information is available from Toxbase: www.spib.axl.co.uk; or the National Poisons Information Service: Tel. 0870 6006266).

Assessment of circulation

There should be no signs of shock in the first 2–3 hours after a burn. Often dressings have been left in place well beyond the 10 minutes or so needed for first aid.

⚠ **Wet dressings frequently cause hypothermia and peripheral shutdown.**

Another cause of shock is associated injury. Go back over the history and call for senior help.

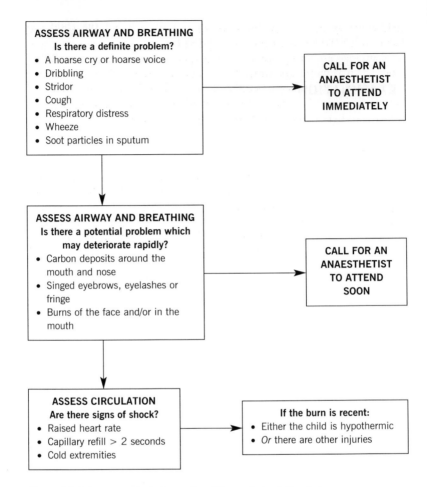

Figure 11.1 Assessment of airway, breathing and circulation in burns.

Depth of burn

(STOP) **Treat pain before making a detailed assessment of the burn itself.**

The depth of burn injury is classified in many ways. 'Superficial' means simply erythema, which fades quickly. Blistered areas are deeper and may be classed sometimes as 'superficial' or more usually as 'partial thickness'. Partial thickness burns are traditionally divided into two categories: 'super-ficial dermal' and 'deep dermal'. The deeper burns are pale and mottled. 'Full thickness' burns appear white, brown or charred, and lack sensation.

In practice, burn depth is difficult to assess in the acute situation and many burns are of mixed depth. If you are unsure, seek advice. At 24–48 hours it is usually much easier to estimate burn severity.

Area of burn

The area of skin that has been injured is expressed as a percentage of the body surface area (BSA). Areas of simple erythema (red skin without blister-ing) are not included in the calculation. The summation of partial thickness and deep areas is done by using the 'rule of nines' as per adult burns charts for post-pubertal children. For younger children, the pattern of burnt areas is drawn on to a modified version of the burns chart (Figure 11.2).

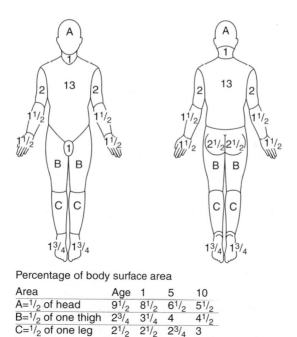

Percentage of body surface area

Area	Age	1	5	10
A=$^1/_2$ of head	$9^1/_2$	$8^1/_2$	$6^1/_2$	$5^1/_2$
B=$^1/_2$ of one thigh	$2^3/_4$	$3^1/_4$	4	$4^1/_2$
C=$^1/_2$ of one leg	$2^1/_2$	$2^1/_2$	$2^3/_4$	3

Figure 11.2 Lund and Browder charts for assessment of burn area in children.

For small areas of burn, a simpler method is to calculate the area using 1% as the area of the child's hand, including the fingers (not just the palm, as commonly misunderstood).

⚠ Check that your findings on examination are compatible with the history given because of possible non-accidental injury (see Chapter 15).

MANAGEMENT OF NON-MAJOR BURNS

First aid treatment

The first aid treatment for minor burn injury is to run cold water over the affected part for 5 minutes or immerse in tepid water. Then cover the wound with a clean non-fluffy dressing or cling wrap.

⚠ Do not leave wet cloths on the burn areas as this can cause hypothermia.

Initially creams or ointments should not be put on the burn. Parents may apply these or other inappropriate substances, such as toothpaste or butter, to the burn. This should be gently discouraged for potential future accidents and the correct first aid advice given.

Pain

⚠ Treat pain before making a detailed assessment of the burn itself.

Pain is always present in minor burn injury because nerve endings in the skin have been damaged and are exposed. Therefore, covering the burn is the best way of soothing pain. Non-pharmacological methods of pain relief should be tried:
• calming the carer and the child;
• covering the injuries with cling wrap or dressings;
• distraction.

Keep the burn covered until the analgesia is working. Usually oral paracetamol plus opiate analgesia, either oral or intranasal, will be adequate for minor burns. Opiates help with anxiolysis. Refer to Chapter 3 'Pain Management'.

If the child will be discharged home, analgesia should be prescribed for at least 24 hours after the injury. In addition, the carer should be asked to give a dose half an hour before the time of the appointment for dressing changes (see 'Follow-up', below).

Specialist referral

Burns that should be referred for same-day specialist advice are those involving more than 10% BSA, any with full thickness areas and those in special areas, e.g. around the eyes, mouth, perineum or napkin area, or nipple.

Dressings

If specialist advice is required (see above), temporary dressings, such as cling wrap are perfectly acceptable. For definitive burn dressing, the wounds should gently be cleaned with water first. Initially, the wounds should be dressed with a non-adherent dressing, such as paraffin gauze. Some departments advocate the use of silver sulphadiazine (Flamazine™), which is soothing but distorts the appearance of the burn. Facial wounds are very difficult to dress so can be left exposed and Vaseline™ ointment applied regularly.

Follow-up

The location of follow-up will depend on local guidelines, but many children with burns should be followed up in a specialist clinic. This may include emergency department clinics, provided there is senior supervision. If complications are unlikely and only simple dressings required, dressing changes may be done by a nursing home care team or at the family doctor's practice.

Dressings such as paraffin gauze (Jelonet™) or silicon-based dressings (Mepitel™) prevent the burn sticking. After the first day or two, dressing changes should be minimized, to avoid disturbing healing tissues.

The length of follow-up will depend on local arrangements. As a rough guide, any burn that takes more than 3 weeks to heal should be reviewed at 6 weeks and at 3 months after healing to check for the development of hypertrophy in the scar. If this occurs, the child should be referred to a specialist.

COMPLICATIONS

Infection

This is rare in the first 48 hours. Infection prevents wound healing but can be difficult to diagnose. Erythema around burns is common and does not need to be treated with systemic antibiotics. You should suspect infection if the burn is painful, the erythema is spreading, the wound has an offensive smell, there is excessive oozing or if the child is systemically unwell (beware toxic shock syndrome, see below).

Mild local infection may clear with daily dressings. If you choose to pre-scribe antibiotics, ensure senior review within 48 hours. Infection should be treated with an anti-Streptococcal and anti-Staphylococcal antibiotic, such as flucloxacillin or erythromycin. Swabs should be taken for microbiologi-cal analysis but the results must be interpreted with caution, since many burns have organisms in the healing tissues.

Toxic shock syndrome

This is much more common in children than adults and can occur in a child with a very minor burn. It usually presents after the first 24 hours and is caused by a toxin-secreting Staphylococcus. Prognosis is related to time to diagnosis, with delay increasing mortality.

The presenting symptoms are fever, rash with shedding of the skin (desquamation) and watery diarrhoea. Clinically the child is shocked and may progress to need intensive care.

STOP Assess A, B, C and start treatment immediately with boluses of intravenous fluid and anti-Staphylococcal antibiotics. Call for senior help and transfer urgently to specialist care.

CHEMICAL INJURIES

General information

Chemical injuries most commonly occur owing to accidents in schools or with cleaning agents in the home. The burnt areas should be thoroughly washed with running water until further facts are established. Specific anti-dotes are rarely necessary but advice should be sought from your local poisons information service (in the UK this information is available from Toxbase: www.spib.axl.co.uk; or the National Poisons Information Service: Tel. 0870 6006266). *For chemical injuries to the eyes, see Chapter 5 'Head and Facial Injuries'.*

Find out if the chemical is acid or alkali by dipping litmus paper into the offending liquid.

⚠ Different types of litmus paper are available. Use the paper that gives you a pH value.

Acids

Acid substances usually cause immediate pain, but most burns are superficial because acids cause coagulation of the surface tissues, thus forming a protective barrier to further damage. Treat by irrigation using 500 ml of saline, via an IV giving set. Repeat if pain is still present.

Alkalis

Alkalis are found in household cleaning products, and may be highly concentrated in substances such as oven cleaner or dishwasher tablets. Wet concrete is also alkaline and, while uncommon as a childhood injury, is very serious.

⚠ Alkaline injuries are much more serious than acid injuries. Obtain senior help.

Alkalis permeate between cell membranes, causing deep-seated damage. Deceptively, they may be less painful than acids initially. Treat by irrigation (as above) but it may take several hours for the burn to become pain-free.

⚠ Litmus paper is not useful for monitoring response to irrigation, unless tested half an hour after irrigation has stopped and the child is symptom free.

The subsequent management of a chemical burn is the same as a thermal burn (see above).

ELECTRICAL INJURIES

General information

Electrical injuries may cause dysrhythmias, deep burns and deep soft tissue damage. Any cardiac dysrhythmia will be apparent from the time of injury so, if the child is in sinus rhythm when first monitored, there is no need for further monitoring.

Domestic electric supply

Young children sustain electrical burns in the home when they poke metal objects into live sockets or they touch live wires. This type of electrical injury (with a relatively low voltage) leads to well-defined areas of full thickness burns at the entry point of the current. There may also be an exit burn. Damage to deeper structures between entry and exit points can result in a compartment syndrome developing (see Chapter 4 'Wounds and Soft Tissue Injuries').

 Ask for senior advice on the management of these injuries.

High-voltage electricity

Injury due to high voltage electricity most commonly occurs when young people play on railways. Occasionally they are injured while climbing pylons. There are likely to be other severe injuries apart from the burn.

STOP Patients who have injuries due to high-voltage electricity may have severe injuries in addition to a major burn.

HEAT ILLNESS

General information

In prolonged exposure to heat from external sources or prolonged exercise, children may develop:
- heat cramps;
- heat exhaustion – irritability, dizziness, headache, nausea;
- heat stroke – temperature over 41°C, shock, coma, convulsions.

These may be associated with sunburn. The cause is fluid loss from sweating, with inadequate replacement of water and salt. Children with cystic fibrosis are at greater risk.

Management

When the core temperature is over 39.5°C clothes should be removed and the child should be sponged with tepid water. A fan of cold air can be used with caution – if the skin is cooled too rapidly then capillary vasoconstriction occurs and the core temperature rises further.

Standard oral rehydration solutions are usually adequate in the early stages. In heat exhaustion and heat stroke, intravenous replacement is needed.

STOP This is a rare and serious condition. Seek senior help.

12

Bites, stings and allergic reactions

BITES IN GENERAL

History

Bites from various animals are quite common in children. Elicit what type of animal bite (including human) has been sustained. The size of the animal is important, as the larger and more powerful its jaws, the more injury to the surrounding soft tissue will have occurred. Although there are more and more exotic pets being kept in UK households in the last few years, general principles of management of a dirty wound apply (see Chapter 4 'Wounds and Soft Tissue Injuries'). For example, ask about the child's tetanus immunization status.

If the patient knows the person or animal, they can be further assessed for risk of specific infections transmitted by the bite.

Examination

Assess the wound for damage to superficial and deep structures, including nerves, vessels, joints and tendons. A powerful bite may break bones.

Management

Consider X-rays if you suspect a fracture or foreign body (ask about the possibility of a broken tooth). The large number of commensal bacteria in an animal's mouth means that all bites are contaminated wounds.

⚠️ **The risk of infection is increased in puncture versus open wounds (see Chapter 4 'Wounds and Superficial Injuries').**

Irrigate and explore the wound thoroughly (see Chapter 17 'Practical Procedures'). Bites are usually left open. However, if the wound is gaping or a good cosmetic result is required, then surgical debridement and closure may be appropriate. Seek senior advice first.

Consider antibiotic prophylaxis:
- if the wound is more than 24 hours old;
- puncture wounds;
- extensive tissue damage;
- wounds to the hands;
- if the wound has been closed.

Administer tetanus immunization or immunoglobulin for high-risk wounds (see Chapter 4 'Wounds and Superficial Injuries'). Consider rabies prophylaxis if the child was bitten outside the British Isles. The rabies status of the animal is usually unknown. In these circumstances, even if the wound is several weeks old, rabies prophylaxis should be given as the rabies virus incubation period is up to 12 weeks.

HUMAN BITES

History

Human bites must always be taken seriously. The human mouth carries large numbers of aerobic and anaerobic bacteria, which means that bites have a high risk of infection. If the person who bit the patient is known to have, or is at risk of, hepatitis or HIV infection, consider whether there may be transmission of the virus. Follow your local guidelines if you think the child is at risk.

⚠️ **Remember the history of a bite may not be clear, for example, a wound from a punch type injury or in non-accidental injury (see Chapter 15).**

Examination

See bites in general.

Management

See bites in general. Prophylactic antibiotics are required to cover both aerobic and anaerobic bacteria, e.g. co-amoxyclavulinic acid. If the child is allergic to penicillin, prescribe erythromycin and metronidazole. Consider hepatitis B and/or HIV prophylaxis (see above).

DOG BITES

History

The child may have been very frightened by the event, and bites from aggressive dogs may involve the police and the Dangerous Dogs Act. The size of dog is important, as a bite from a large dog is associated with significant soft tissue and bone injury.

Examination

See bites in general.

Management

See bites in general.

CAT BITES

History

See bites in general.

Examination

See bites in general.

Management

See bites in general. The most common organism to cause infection is *Pasteurella multocida*, which is found as a commensal in the mouths of cats.

This can lead to severe wound sepsis with associated septicaemia. Penicillin is the antibiotic of choice for *Pasteurella*. If allergic to penicillin, prescribe erythromycin, although this is less effective.

RAT BITES

History

Establish whether the rat is a pet or was wild. Wild rats can transmit leptospirosis (Weil's disease).

Examination

See bites in general.

Management

See bites in general. Give prophylactic penicillin. If the child is allergic to penicillin, doxycycline can be give as an alternative if the child is over 12 years. For younger children prescribe erythromycin.

SNAKE BITES

History

Try to identify the snake. The only poisonous snake native to the British Isles is the adder (*Vipera berus*). Adder bites generally only lead to local symptoms. More serious bites from imported snakes (envenomation) are occasionally seen. Systemic symptoms include respiratory distress, vomiting, abdominal pain or diarrhoea.

Examination

Local effects include pain, swelling, bruising and enlargement of regional lymph nodes. Systemic signs of envenoming are hypotension, angioedema, depressed level of consciousness, electrocardiogram (ECG) abnormalities, spontaneous bleeding, coagulopathy, respiratory distress and acute renal failure.

Management

If the bite is on a limb, the whole limb should be bandaged with a compression bandage and immobilized to reduce systemic effects. Do not apply a tourniquet.

 If any signs of envenomation: assess A, B, C.

⚠ **Ask senior advice and consult your local poisons information centre for further management.** (In the UK this information is available from Toxbase: www.spib.axl.co.uk; or the National Poisons Information Service: Tel. 0870 6006266.)

INSECT BITES

Bites may occur without a clear history. Symptoms within the first 48 hours are caused by a localized allergic response causing itching, erythema and swelling. After this time, erythema and swelling may indicate secondary bacterial infection.

Management

Ice packs, elevation and analgesia can give symptomatic relief. If further treatment is needed, advise topical and/or oral antihistamines. If secondary bacterial infection is suspected, then give oral antibiotic, e.g. flucloxacillin.

STINGS

Bee and wasp stings

Rarely, a sting may lead to a generalized severe anaphylactic response in a susceptible individual (see below). However, bee and wasp stings more usually present as localized pain and swelling.

If the sting is still present, remove it from the skin. Treat as for insect bites.

Jellyfish stings

Stings from jellyfish in the waters around the British Isles lead to local irritation only. Treat as for insect bites.

ALLERGIC REACTIONS

History

Allergic reactions vary from mild to severe. The speed of progression of symptoms is a guide to severity. Severe reactions usually occur within 2–20 minutes of exposure. Peanut and latex allergies are becoming more common. In the context of injuries, enquiries must be made concerning allergy to dressings, tetanus immunization and antibiotics.

Examination

Symptoms and signs can be localized or systemic. They can be mild, moderate or severe, and may affect the following:
- the airway and mouth – lip, tongue and mouth swelling, difficulty; swallowing or speaking, stridor;
- breathing – difficulty in breathing, wheezing;
- circulation – flushing, peripheral vasodilation, hypotension;
- skin – flushing, urticaria, sweating;
- gastrointestinal tract – nausea, diarrhoea, abdominal pain.

For moderate or severe reactions, you should have a low threshold for administration of intramuscular adrenaline.

(STOP) **If symptoms are severe – get help. Remove the allergen! Give epinephrine 10 mg/kg intramuscularly. Treat A, B, C – see APLS guidelines.**

Management

See Figure 12.1.

ASSESS AIRWAY, BREATHING AND CIRCULATION

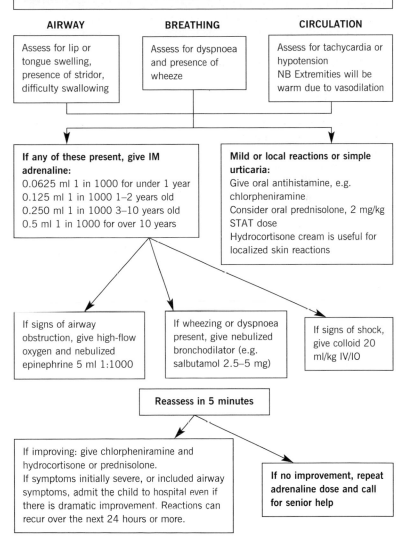

Figure 12.1 Treatment of allergic reactions.

Foreign bodies

SOFT TISSUES

Presentation to the emergency department with a foreign body (FB) is very common, occurring either through injury or deliberately (usually young children). Your management will depend upon:
- the site;
- the size;
- the presence or absence of infection;
- the length of time the FB has been there;
- the nature of the FB.

 It is important to do no further harm.

Site

Think before you try to remove a FB. For instance, are you in dangerous territory, such as near vessels or important nerves? Might you need to extend a wound? If so, is it safe to do so?

 If in doubt, refer to a surgeon.

FBs in body cavities must be removed, as well as those in the eye, in a joint, over pressure areas, such as the elbow, and in those sites listed specifically below.

For further information about FBs in wounds, see Chapter 4 'Wounds and Soft Tissue Injuries'.

Size

If the FB requires a large anaesthetic field for its removal, calculate the maximum safe dose of anaesthetic you may use, for the size of the child (see Chapter 17 'Practical Procedures'). If you are likely to exceed this dose, refer for general anaesthesia. Might you have to extend the wound? (see above).

Infection

If infection is present (cellulitis or abscess), the FB is likely to need to be removed. This situation is more complex and you should ask for senior advice.

Duration

If the wound has closed (24–48 hours), even a FB that looks superficial on X-ray may be very difficult to remove. Unless it is easily palpable under the skin, refer to a surgeon.

Nature of the FB

Organic FBs are more likely to cause infections and other complications, whereas some inorganic FBs, such as small pieces of glass or airgun pellets, can remain *in situ* for life, or at least many years, before causing problems.

Splinters

These are commonly found in hands or under nails (refer also to 'Hand – General Principles' on p. 91). Splinters should be removed using 'splinter forceps'. These are a special kind of forceps with a very fine point – always use them, as they make removal much easier.

Small pieces of splinter or dirt remaining far under the nail after the main splinter has been removed should be left alone – most wood softens to a pulp in a few days and will come out with a bead of pus.

Fish hooks

These are usually embedded in fingers. There are three methods of removal, depending on the size of the barb. Small barbs may simply be pulled out, although an incision may be necessary to enlarge the wound.

Those with a single barb close to the shaft may be pulled out with an 18- or 16-gauge needle inserted on to the tip of the barb, to 'cover' it and stop it sticking on the way out.

Larger barbs may have to be 'pushed through'. The shaft is fed into the finger until the barb starts to cause bulging of the overlying skin. A scalpel is then used to create an exit point for the barb, then the whole thing is fed through this new incision.

Glass

⚠ **Always request a soft tissue X-ray for wounds caused by glass.**

Glass can be very difficult to find in a wound. Most glass is radio-opaque. Once the FB has been removed, a confirmatory X-ray is imperative.

Ultrasound

Soft tissue ultrasound is a good method of identifying the presence of a foreign body if exploration and X-rays are negative, but you still have a high index of suspicion. The accuracy of ultrasound depends on operator experience and should be discussed with a radiologist.

THE EYE

See Chapter 5 'Head and Facial Injuries'.

THE EAR

External auditory canal

History
This is very common in young children. The child may present with a history of inserting a FB into their ear or may have been witnessed inserting a FB. In others there is no clear history of a FB, and the child presents with pain, deafness or discharge from the ear. Occasionally live insects can enter the ear.

It is often quite a painful condition, and to permit examination or removal the child may need, for example, intranasal diamorphine for both analgesia and anxiolysis (see Chapter 3 'Pain Management').

Examination
The diagnosis of FB requires direct visualization with an auroscope. See Chapter 17 'Practical Procedures'.

Management
See Chapter 17 'Practical Procedures'.

Embedded earrings

Stud-type earrings can become embedded within the pinna. Most commonly, the back or 'butterfly' becomes embedded with inflammation and sometimes infection. If swelling is severe, the front of the earring may also become embedded.

Management
The earring is usually easily removed once adequate pain relief with local anaesthetic is instituted. An inferior auricular nerve block is invaluable (see Chapter 17 'Practical Procedures'). Once pain free, apply gentle pressure to the front of the earring to release the butterfly at the back. Occasionally, a small skin incision over the butterfly is required. Remove the whole earring. If the pinna is infected, antibiotics may be required, although simply removing the earring is often sufficient.

THE NOSE

History

This is very common in young children. The child may present with a history of inserting a FB into their nose or may have been witnessed inserting a FB. In others there is no clear history of a FB, and the child presents with a unilateral, offensive discharge or bleeding from the nose.

Examination

The diagnosis of FB requires direct visualization. Use the same position as for throat examination (see Chapter 17 'Practical Procedures').

Management

Before instrumentation, try the 'kissing' technique (see Chapter 17 'Practical Procedures'.

THE THROAT

History

Usually the child will have ingested something sharp, such as a bone, and have felt it become 'stuck'. Another common situation is that a child has tried to swallow a coin.

⚠ **If there is any history of choking, consider inhalation (see below).**

Examination

⚠ **If the child is distressed, call for senior help! Do not upset the child further, or send him or her for an X-ray.**

The majority of children are able to describe their symptoms, and in most cases the FB is a bone. It has often descended into the stomach and it is the scratch caused by the bone that is still felt.

Examine the throat (see Chapter 17 'Practical Procedures') and, if it cannot be seen, it may be behind the fauces, on the tonsil. If the child will cooperate, spray the throat with lignocaine anaesthetic, use a tongue depressing spatula to push the anterior fauces to one side and the bone may come into view.

Management

If the FB is visualized, remove it with small Magill's or Tilley's forceps. If examination of the mouth does not reveal a FB, consider whether it is radioopaque and will, therefore, be seen on a soft tissue lateral neck X-ray.

Fish bones may or may not show up, depending on the size and type of bone. They can roughly be divided into those that are and are not visible by this silly *aide memoire*: 'main courses' do (e.g. plaice or cod) and 'starters' do not (e.g. kippers, mackerel, salmon and trout)! If in doubt, ask your radiographer.

If the FB is visible in the hypopharynx or oesophagus on X-ray, refer to the ear, nose and throat (ENT or otolaryngology) specialists. If the FB has not shown up on X-ray or is not radio-opaque, your management depends on the degree of distress. If distressed refer to the ENT specialists. However, the majority of children can go home with simple analgesia, be encouraged to drink and eat soft foods, and attend an outpatient clinic 24 hours later if symptoms persist – symptoms of a scratch will be improving at this stage.

INHALED FOREIGN BODIES

Inhaled foreign body occurs most commonly in pre-school children. Almost anything can be inhaled and foodstuffs, such as peanuts or sweets, or beads are the commonest offending items. Sadly, inhaled FBs causing severe airway obstruction often result in death at home or *en route* to hospital.

The history of inhaled FB is not always clear, unless witnessed, but sudden onset of airway symptoms in a child who was previously well is strongly suggestive of an inhaled FB. Sometimes it may present several weeks or months later, and can be mistaken for asthma.

Upper airway

As described above, children with complete airway obstruction rarely survive to hospital. There is most likely to be stridor, gagging, choking or drooling, but sometimes the child may just be very quiet and apprehensive, and sitting in a posture in which they are most comfortable. If this is the case, it is imperative not to upset the child further. Crying and struggling may convert a partially obstructed airway into a completely obstructed one.

STOP Proceed to a resuscitation area but keep the child as calm as possible.

Encourage and reassure the child while awaiting senior help. Use the time to prepare equipment such as Magill's forceps, equipment for intubation and needle cricothyroidotomy.

An algorithm for upper airway obstruction is presented in Figure 13.1. The algorithm for back blows, the Heimlich manoeuvre and chest thrusts is shown in Figure 13.2. These manoeuvres are demonstrated in Figures 13.3–13.5.

It is important to differentiate FB from other causes of stridor, as any attempts at manoeuvres to remove a FB may completely obstruct the airway of a child with an infective cause of stridor.

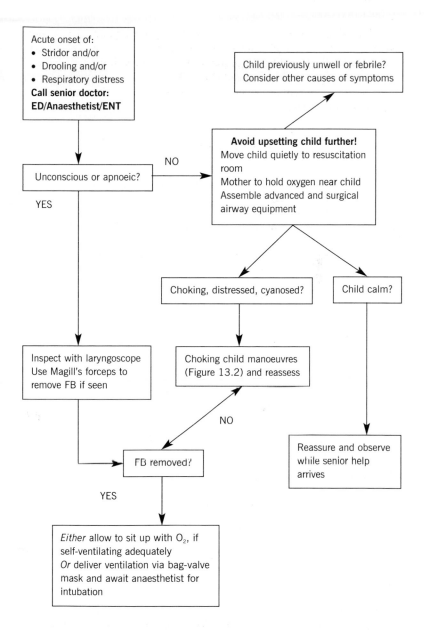

Figure 13.1 Management of an inhaled foreign body (FB) in the upper airway.

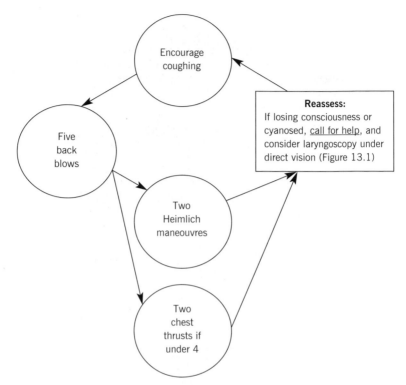

Figure 13.2 Management of the choking child.

Lower airway

Acutely, a child will present with persistent cough or wheeze. On examination, localized breath sounds may be absent and/or wheeze may be present. However, examination may be normal.

⚠ Beware delayed presentation.

Children can present with signs of wheezing, a pneumonia or empyema with no history of an inhaled foreign body.

Investigations

A chest X-ray should be performed. If the FB is radio-opaque, it may be visible. In 90% of acute cases there is hyperinflation of the lung distal to the

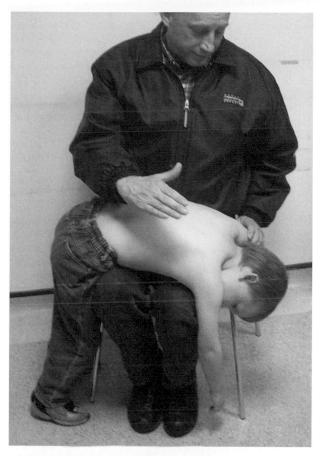

Figure 13.3 Back blows.

FB, which can act as a ball valve, allowing air to enter but not be expelled from the obstructed segment (Figure 13.6). In the remainder (particularly with a delay in presentation or diagnosis) there are signs of collapse of the obstructed segment of lung.

Management
Refer for removal of FB by bronchoscopy under general anaesthesia.

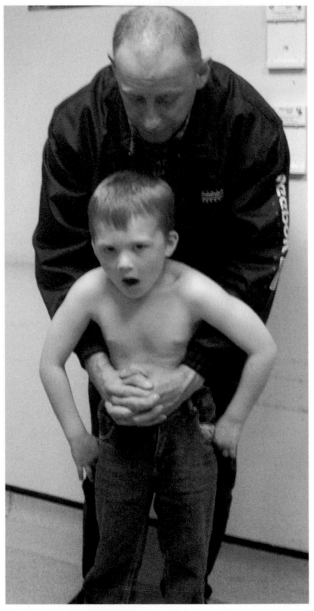

Figure 13.4 The Heimlich manoeuvre.

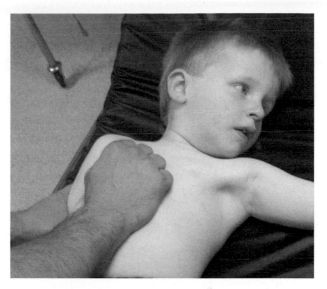

Figure 13.5 Chest thrusts in the young child.

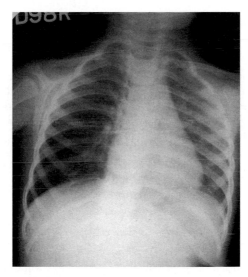

A

Figure 13.6 Chest X-ray demonstrating lung hyperinflation of right lung (due to 'ball-valve effect') after inhalation of a foreign body.

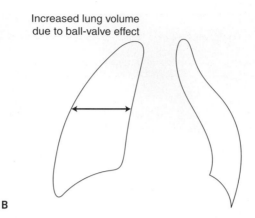

Increased lung volume
due to ball-valve effect

B

Figure 13.6 *continued.*

SWALLOWED FOREIGN BODIES

History

For foreign bodies in the throat, see above.

Ingestion of a foreign body is common in children. The child may give a history of ingestion or be witnessed swallowing a FB. The parent or carer may give a history of items last seen with the child now being missing, or alternatively the child may be found retching or choking.

⚠ **In a child with a 'swallowed' foreign body, ask specifically for coughing.**

Coughing is a good clue that it may be in the airway (see 'Inhaled foreign bodies', above).

Management

Provided they reach the stomach, most ingested FBs will pass through the gastrointestinal tract uneventfully (see Figure 13.7). If requesting an X-ray, ask for a 'mouth to upper abdomen' X-ray.

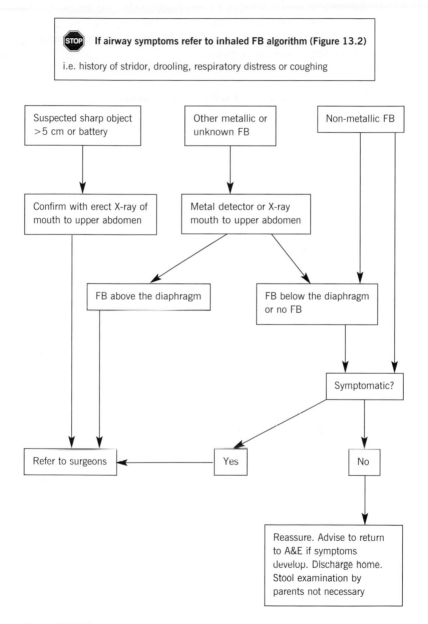

Figure 13.7 Management of a swallowed foreign body (FB).

If discharging the child, advise the parents that complications are very unlikely, but that they should return if the child starts vomiting, refusing to eat or complaining of abdominal pain.

VAGINAL AND RECTAL FOREIGN BODIES

History

A vaginal or rectal foreign body is rare in younger children and there is often no clear history. The child will usually present with discharge or pain. Although simple experimentation occurs, inappropriate sexualized behaviour should be considered.

(STOP) Consider sexual abuse and seek senior help (see Chapter 15).

Adolescent girls may present with a history of a lost tampon or a lost condom.

Management

All young children with suspected vaginal or rectal FB should be referred for further specialist assessment. It is not appropriate to perform a vaginal or rectal examination of a young child in the emergency department.

In adolescents, removal of a lost tampon or other vaginal FB is often simple. If the FB is a lost condom or other sexual item, remember to consider the maturity of the girl, the appropriateness or consensuality of the sexual liaison, and issues such as post-coital contraception and sexually transmitted diseases (refer if necessary to Chapter 15 'Non-accidental Injury' and Chapter 16 'Medicolegal and Forensic Issues'). Seek senior help if you are unsure.

Injuries of the external genitalia and anus

INTRODUCTION

Injury to the genital area is rare under the age of 2 years. Trauma in this area becomes more likely as children become mobile and increase their ranges of activities. Accidental anal injury is rare at all ages.

 Remember the possibility of non-accidental injury (see Chapter 15).

There is obviously a great deal of psychological distress associated with injuries in this area. Most children presenting to the emergency department have bled immediately after the incident. This alarms parents but fortunately most have stopped bleeding by the time they reach hospital.

Many injuries cause pain and this is very severe as the genital area has a rich nerve supply (see Chapter 3 'Pain Management'). Some children have discomfort on passing urine at presentation and blood in the urine. This is rarely from the urethra, usually being contamination by blood from the injured genitalia.

From about 4 years old, children can be embarrassed or anxious about examination of the area. It is important to look calm, be reassuring and examine children in privacy. It is wise to involve another doctor or nurse, if you feel inexperienced in examining this area, to avoid repeated examination of the child.

When examining the female genitalia, be precise when describing the injured areas (Figure 14.1).

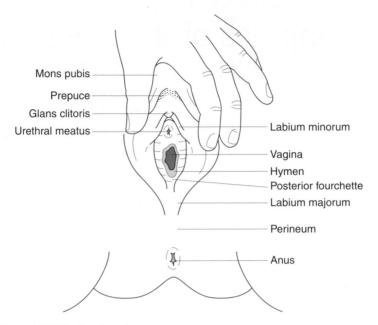

Figure 14.1 The female perineum.

FEMALE EXTERNAL GENITAL INJURIES

Blunt injury

A fall on to a hard object, particularly a straddle-type injury, such as astride the bath or gym equipment, is the commonest cause of injury to female external genitalia. The direct force involved leads to compression of the soft tissues of the vulva between the object and the pelvis. This causes bruising, abrasions and/or lacerations, which are usually anterior and asymmetrical. Lacerations usually tend to be superficial, and are most commonly found between the labia majora and labia minora. Bruising of the soft tissues may be severe but the hymen is not damaged. A punch or kick to the genital area gives similar findings to a fall on to a hard object. This assault may be unintentional in rough play. If there is any suspicion that the injury was intentional, refer to your local child protection policy and Chapter 15 'Non-accidental Injury'.

Clean all abrasions and superficial lacerations thoroughly with normal saline. Leave them exposed. Advise frequent warm saline baths or very gentle showering of the affected area, avoiding soap. Most will heal within a week. Advise the parents to ensure frequent analgesia, if necessary, and encouragement of oral fluids so that weak urine is passed frequently, so as to avoid urinary retention.

Stretch injuries

When females accidentally do 'the splits', this can result in superficial lacerations of the skin of the perineum or posterior fourchette, especially if labial adhesions are present. Management is as described above.

Accidental penetrating injury

This mechanism is less common but potentially more damaging. Make sure that the full depth of penetration can be visualized. If superficial, manage as above. If not, refer to an experienced surgeon.

 Some of these injuries are deceptively deep and require surgical exploration and repair.

MALE EXTERNAL GENITAL INJURIES

Penile blunt injury

Most penile injuries in childhood are due to a fall on to a hard surface or an object falling on to the penis. These result in contusions and superficial lacerations.

⚠ Beware of a large haematoma following minor trauma – this could be a ruptured *corpus cavernosus*, which needs surgical exploration.

Clean all abrasions and superficial lacerations thoroughly with normal saline. Leave them exposed. Advise frequent warm baths or very gentle showering of the affected area, avoiding soap. Most will heal within a week. Advise the parents to ensure frequent analgesia, if necessary, and encouragement of oral fluids so that weak urine is passed frequently, so as to avoid urinary retention.

Zipper injury

The foreskin or shaft of the penis may get caught in a zipper, causing an abrasion or superficial laceration. The zipper can be disengaged by cutting its distal end off and separating the two halves. A penile block is relatively straightforward – ask for senior advice. A sedative analgesic, such as intranasal diamorphine, or conscious sedation, or sometimes general anaesthesia, may be necessary (see Chapter 3 'Pain Management').

Strangulation injury

A variety of objects (e.g. hair, fibres from clothes, rubber bands) may be put accidentally or intentionally around the penis. The object acts as a tourniquet and the penis becomes swollen distal to the tight band. As the swelling increases, the constricting band can become buried and invisible. Urgent release of the constriction is necessary. Try to remove the constricting object by unwinding it from the penis. If this is not possible, then surgical exploration and removal under general anaesthesia will be needed.

🛑 **If the condition is not diagnosed promptly, tissue loss may occur.**

Injuries to the scrotum and testes

A punch or kick gives similar findings to a fall on to a hard object. This may be unintentional in rough play. If there is any suspicion that it was intentional, follow your local child protection policy and refer to Chapter 15 'Non-accidental Injury'.

The most likely injury is a contusion. The resultant swelling may make it difficult to decide whether this is a simple contusion or whether the testis has been damaged. An ultrasound examination will be helpful if injury to the testis is suspected. All penetrating injuries to the scrotum or testes caused by sharp objects must be referred to an experienced surgeon.

ANAL INJURIES

Minor injury to the anus owing to an accident in childhood is very uncommon. Anal fissures can occur in the constipated child passing a hard stool.

All patients with anal and perianal injuries should be referred for senior advice.

ASSOCIATED PATHOLOGY

Sometimes minor trauma can cause more severe effects, if the area was already inflamed. This will potentially confuse your examination. Examples of such conditions include vulvovaginitis, psoriasis, streptococcal infection, candidiasis, threadworms, lichen sclerosis et atrophicus or inflammatory bowel disease.

SELF-INFLICTED INJURIES

Self-inflicted injury is unlikely except in children with learning disabilities. If a parent alleges, or the child confesses, that an injury was self-inflicted, senior advice should be sought.

⚠ Deliberate self-harm must be taken seriously and a full psychosocial assessment performed by an experienced multidisciplinary team.

Minor abrasions can occur if children scratch themselves because of irritation owing to vulvovaginitis or threadworms. These conditions commonly occur under the age of 6 years.

DIFFERENTIATION BETWEEN ACCIDENTAL INJURY AND ASSAULT

 If you are at all suspicious about physical or sexual assault, follow your local child protection policy.

In the context of a history of injury, these situations are uncommon, since the vast majority of injuries are perfectly innocent. However, you must seek senior advice if you are at all unsure. As well as the indicators of non-accidental injury described in Chapter 15, suspect physical or sexual assault of the external genital or anus if your findings are incompatible with the history given, based on the classical types of injury pattern described above, or if there is any evidence of a sexually transmitted disease.

Physical signs of injury are rare in sexually abused female children. Fingering may cause abrasions. The classical injury in attempted penile penetration involves a thrust directed posteriorly, which first tears the fourchette and then the hymen and posterior wall of the vagina. Laceration occurs with little bruising.

Symmetrical small bruises on the penis may be due to a pinch.

Further reading

1. Most textbooks of paediatric surgery.
2. Garden A S (editor): *Paediatric and adolescent gynaecology.* London: Arnold, 1998.

Non-accidental injury

INTRODUCTION

Sadly, any clinician treating minor injuries in children has to be aware of the possibility of non-accidental injury. You could be forgiven for thinking that paediatricians are perhaps obsessed by the subject but the reality is that delay in diagnosis is still common, the diagnosis itself can be extremely difficult to make, and the repercussions of either a 'false-negative' or 'false-positive' diagnosis can be very damaging.

(STOP) **Remember that the first non-accidental injury may be minor trauma, but that abuse may escalate until morbidity or death results.**

If non-accidental injury (NAI) is suspected, a full assessment of the infant or child must be done by a doctor who is trained in that field. Nearly all hospitals or minor injury units have local policies for suspected NAI.

(STOP) **Follow your local child protection policy at all times.**

THE SPECTRUM OF CHILD ABUSE

The Child Protection Register is held at local authority level. Some emergency departments have 24-hour access to it. However, remember that there may be many injuries inflicted before a diagnosis of NAI is made. The categories of abuse include not only physical abuse, but also neglect, emotional abuse and sexual abuse.

Statistically, physical abuse is more common in the under 2-year-old age group, and is associated with social fragmentation. However, it occurs in all social classes and at all ages. As well as intentional injury, neglect and poor supervision are common causes of presentation to the emergency department (see Chapters 1 and 2). However, this is a difficult judgement to make, especially if a family is living in overcrowded, poor accommodation.

TYPES OF NON-ACCIDENTAL INJURY

The 'battered baby syndrome' and the 'shaken baby syndrome' are overlapping clinical pictures where occult injury may be present. Examples of such injuries are:
- subdural and extradural haemorrhage (see below and Chapter 5);
- spiral fractures of the humerus (Chapter 8) or femur (Chapter 10);
- fractured ribs.

You may be presented with one injury, such as a limb fracture, when in fact several are present. The presence of retinal haemorrhages strongly supports this diagnosis, although these are often difficult to see in an irritable infant.

Above this age, inflicted injuries can be difficult to distinguish from non-intentional injury.

POINTERS TO NON-ACCIDENTAL INJURY

⚠ **At any time in your consultation there may be a pointer to NAI.**

General

Suspect NAI in the following circumstances:
- the story of the 'accident' is vague and lacks detail;
- the story is variable and changes with each telling, e.g. to the nurse, to the doctor, in radiology;
- there has been a delay in seeking medical help;
- the history is not compatible with the injury observed;
- there have been many previous attendances with injuries or minor medical conditions;
- there is a history of injury due to violence in other family members;

- the child discloses abuse (this is unusual);
- the appearance of the child and/or the interaction with the carers appears abnormal.

Injury in an infant who is not fully mobile

 Injuries in the non-mobile infant are uncommon and must raise the suspicion of NAI.

Injuries occurring in babies and infants not yet walking independently are unusual. This is because mobility is very limited at these developmental stages. Most infants are constantly supervised unless placed in a safe place. It is, therefore, unusual, for example, for an infant incapable of rolling to fall off a bed.

⚠ **Be highly suspicious of injury with no explanation.**

Examples of typical non-intentional injuries are:
- the baby is in a baby bouncer or car seat, inappropriately left on a high surface;
- the baby is in a babywalker, unsupervised, and falls off a step or down stairs;
- the baby is dropped or the carer fell when holding the infant.

⚠ **Always consider whether the stated mechanism is likely in terms of the infant's stage of development.**

Most trauma in this age group justifies an X-ray because of poor protective reflexes, difficulty in clinical examination and the possibility of a false history of the mechanism of injury.

Pointers to a significant head injury in an infant include:
- the child is jittery;
- the child is irritable;
- the child is reluctant to feed;
- apnoeic episodes;
- drowsiness;
- persistent vomiting.

These symptoms require a CT scan (see Chapter 5 'Head and Facial Injuries'). There may be little external evidence of injury.

⚠ **Injury to the brain is the commonest cause of death in physical abuse.**

A CT will be helpful in establishing the diagnosis of the shaken baby syndrome.

WHAT DO I DO IF I HAVE CONCERNS?

🛑 **Follow your local child protection policy at all times.**

The assessment of NAI is a multiagency one. If you are unsure, you have a professional duty to raise the concerns you may have, but it is not usually your responsibility to make a judgement about whether this injury is accidental or intentional. Do not be worried about alerting the system: it will not have dramatic effects and you will not be held responsible for decisions taken. Most areas have skilled personnel who are able to assess the risk to the child and who do not act hastily.

Before you say or do anything, check the registration information with the carer before leaving the room. This means:

- their full name;
- the child's up-to-date address and how long they have been there;
- any other names by which the child may be known;
- the child's date of birth;
- their contact telephone number;
- their relationship to the child;
- any recent previous address;
- the names of their family doctor and health visitor.

These facts will help significantly if the family subsequently absconds.

Next, your local child protection policy is likely to first suggest a full medical assessment by an experienced paediatrician. The best way to phrase this to the family is to say that you are inexperienced in such injuries, and would like advice from a specialist children's doctor, as it is important that this injury is treated correctly from the beginning. It is difficult for the family to be annoyed about this.

THE CHILD PROTECTION SYSTEM

In parallel with the above, the Child Protection Register will be checked by the area or duty social worker. Remember that the check is only a small part of the assessment – names and addresses change, updating takes time and children on the register do have accidents! The health visitor for the family will also be contacted early for information on the family dynamics. The health visitor can be contacted via the family doctor's practice.

Full multiagency assessment involves a wide variety of professional people who have had contact with the family, such as teachers, police officers and social workers. A strategy meeting will probably take place, and includes the parents and other carers.

Each person will bring his or her knowledge of the family to a case discussion or case conference. You are unlikely to be invited to such a meeting – it is more likely to be the paediatrician involved in the case. Decisions will then be made on the future care of all children in the family.

Further reading

1. Department of Health: *Working together to safeguard children*. London: Department of Health, 1999.
2. Meadow R (ed.): *ABC of child abuse*. London: BMJ Publishing, 1997.

Medicolegal and forensic issues

INTRODUCTION

This chapter is not an exhaustive text, but a guide for those practising in the emergency department. If you practise outside England and Wales, please seek senior advice on any of these issues. The law is different in each country, although many of the principles are around basic professional practice, as outlined in the General Medical Council's 'Good Medical Practice' guide and its other publications.

CONSENT

When do I need consent?

Doctors should rarely need to consult patients against their will. However, failure to obtain consent may lead to disciplinary proceedings for professional misconduct, or civil action for damages or criminal proceedings for assault. Consent may be obtained from the legal guardian (see below) or the child, if they are competent (see below).

In paediatric practice, the most likely scenario you will face is a child objecting to examination or a procedure, which in most cases is easily over-come with experience. Common sense is essential and it stands to reason that certain sensitive procedures, such as intimate examinations, particu-larly of a young girl by a male clinician, require another member of staff as a chaperone. On occasion, however, a working knowledge of the law is essential.

Implied consent
Routine doctor/patient interaction does not require specific consent, since consent is implied by voluntarily attendance for consultation.

Express consent
More specific consent should be sought, if examination involves invasion of the body cavities or the handling of the external genitalia or if a procedure needs to be performed. Express consent may be verbal or in writing. For small procedures, such as suturing, written consent is not normally sought in the UK; beyond this, individual practice varies but written consent should be sought if the procedure entails clouding of consciousness (e.g. for conscious sedation). Ideally, oral expressed consent should be witnessed by a third party.

Who is a legal guardian?

If a child is legitimate (i.e. the parents are married at the time of birth or are married at any time since conception), each parent can consent separately. If the child is illegitimate, the mother always has parental responsibility and can, therefore, give consent. The unmarried father can acquire parental responsibility:

- by marrying the mother;
- by applying to court for a parental responsibility order;
- by former agreement with the mother;
- by being appointed guardian by the mother or the court on the death of the mother;
- by obtaining a residence order under Section 8 of the Children Act.

Other legal guardians are appointed by the court, and may be other family members, a foster parent, the police or a social worker. You must be very clear whether such persons are official legal guardians.

When is a child competent?

Below the age of 16, in accordance with the Children Act, 1989, a young per-son may give his/her own permission, if they are sufficiently mature to be aware of the purposes of the examination, and to understand the treatment being recommended (Gillick competence).

A more recent legal definition of competence is that the person must:

(a) understand the concept the doctor/nurse is explaining and have the memory to retain that information;

(b) be able to balance the consequences of treatment versus non-treatment; and

(c) believe that information to be true.

If there is any doubt about the patient's ability to understand the nature of the examination or proposed procedures, consent should be obtained from their legal guardian (see above). If this is not possible, it is good practice to involve another family member, although in legal terms they are unable to give consent.

What if I cannot obtain consent?

If you are unable to obtain consent, (e.g. from an unconscious child or a child not competent to give their own consent, see above), it is wise to wait for their legal guardian; however, you may treat under common law if it is an emergency. In practice, it is common for a child to be brought by another family member or a teacher, and, while caution should be exercised, clinical examination and X-rays are commonly performed in good faith.

What if consent is refused?

In situations where the child is competent, but his/her opinion is contrary to medical opinion, the child's wish may be overturned by someone with parental responsibility, as defined above (except in Scotland), or a doctor. Preferably two doctors, of the most senior grade available, should assess the situation independently, then document their reasons why intervention is in the best interests of the child.

In situations where the legal guardian refuses, you must act in the best interests of the child. If the situation is an emergency, again it is good practice for two doctors to take this decision, as above, and treat under common law. If it is not an emergency, the case must be brought before a court.

What about children with mental disorder, or under the influence of drugs or alcohol?

The ability of a person, who is suffering from a mental disorder or under the influence of drugs or alcohol, to give informed consent must be individually assessed using the three 'tests' described above. The time you spend assessing this depends on the urgency of the situation (as above). A child can be 'sectioned' under the Mental Health Act, but this is usually a lengthy process even in the emergency situation and only provides for psychiatric treatment.

What about written reports?

For written reports of any description (letters to housing authorities, social services, police statements, legal reports, etc.), consent must be provided in writing by the child, if competent, or their legal guardian, unless confidentiality can be broken (see below).

What about forensic specimens?

All forensic specimens should be taken by a police surgeon, who will determine whether consent is or is not necessary (see 'forensic aspects of injuries').

CONFIDENTIALITY

Children are as entitled to confidentiality as adults. It is particularly important to reassure teenagers of this if they are trying to share a problem with you. Confidentiality may be overridden:
• with the patient's consent;
• if there is a threat to the safety of other people;
• if requested to do so by a judge;
• for notifiable diseases.
• for release of information relating to child protection issues to other health professionals on a 'need to know' basis (see *Working Together to Safeguard Children*, published by the Department of Health, 1999);
• under the Road Traffic Act, which permits you to give basic, demographic details about the (suspected) driver;
• under the Prevention of Terrorism Act.

Beware of innocent-sounding requests, which may involve legal battles between, for example, separated parents or housing authorities.

Telephone enquiries

Telephone information should be very basic. Any telephone calls about the patient ideally should be recorded on the definitive records. All requests for detailed information should be made in person or in writing, when more information as to this person's status may be sought.

RECORDS

Contemporaneous notes must be made for every consultation. These must be retained until the patient reaches the age of 25 years. The following is a guide to the information that should be recorded for every child with minor trauma.

Registration details

- name;
- date of birth;
- age;
- permanent address;
- temporary address;
- name and address of next of kin;
- educational establishment;
- general practitioner's name and address.

Nurse assessment

- name of nurse;
- person(s) accompanying the child and their relationship(s) to the child;
- time of assessment;
- triage category (if appropriate);
- pain score;
- relevant vital signs;
- investigations ordered.

Consultation with doctor

- name of doctor;
- date and time of the start of consultation;
- person(s) accompanying the child and their relationship(s) to the child;
- history of present complaint – this must include details of the time of injury, mechanism of injury, any third party involved in the injury and others present;
- history of previous injuries;
- history of intercurrent medical illnesses;
- personal history – medication, allergies, immunizations;

- examination – side, site, shape and size of every injury – diagrams/charts should be used whenever possible;
- investigations and results;
- diagnosis or differential diagnosis;
- management;
- result(s) of investigations performed;
- discharge time and instructions (verbal or written);
- summary letter to general practitioner (copied to health visitor for pre-school children).

If abnormal investigation results are received after discharge from the emergency department, the action taken must be recorded, including the date and time. If the diagnosis was 'missed' (e.g. abnormal X-ray results), follow the same principles as below, and ensure that the family doctor has been informed.

WHAT IF I HAVE MADE A MISTAKE?

(STOP) If you ever realize you have made a clinical mistake, discuss this immediately with a senior doctor.

If the patient's family is still in the department, the senior doctor will give an explanation, apologize and determine if treatment needs to be changed. This rapid local resolution is the best option and is usually accepted by the family. If the patient has gone home, the consultant will make contact, if appropriate, and will probably review the patient in order to apologize and rectify the error, whenever this is possible. Write a full report of the incident and keep a copy.

THE NHS COMPLAINTS SYSTEM

If apologies and an honest explanation are given at the time, or anxious/aggressive situations diffused, complaints are much less likely to happen. This is called 'local resolution'. If a complaint does occur, it will be dealt with by the UK National Health Service hospital complaints system. In brief, your consultant will respond in writing within 20 working days (the letter goes out from the chief executive to the complainant), during which time they will gather information, which will involve asking you for your account of events. If legal action is threatened in the complainant's initial letter, a separate process occurs.

FORENSIC ASPECTS OF INJURIES

General principles

Forensic medicine is a broad field in which medicine comes into relation with the law. Minor trauma in a child may result from a criminal act or may lead to civil proceedings. Sometimes the child or young person with minor trauma is an alleged offender. In all these circumstances, the prime responsibility of the physician or nurse who first sees the child is to assess and treat the child as a patient. This person in addition should do the following.

- Keep accurate contemporaneous records – this must include diagrams with detailed descriptions of every injury, their anatomical positions and measurements. Photographs are invaluable in such situations, although consent for photography should be sought.
- Preserve potential evidence.
- Cooperate with any police and/or social services investigation, but *not release information without consent*, apart from certain circumstances ('Consent and confidentiality').
- If a police officer wishes to question a child, ensure that their medical needs have been met and that the child is appropriately supported (the police have guidelines on interviewing minors).
- If specimens such as blood are required purely for forensic purposes, they should be taken by a police surgeon. Some departments have a policy of allowing emergency department staff to take the specimen, if the patient consents, and it is handed directly to a police officer.

⚠️ Forensic issues can be complex. Always ask for advice from someone with more experience if you are in doubt.

Types of injuries

Abrasions
An abrasion is a superficial graze of the skin.

Bruises (contusions)
A bruise is due to the application of blunt force. The blow ruptures small blood vessels beneath the skin and blood escapes into the surrounding tissues.

Different types of bruises are recognized:
- *petechiae* are pinpoint haemorrhages due to rupture of capillaries caused by shearing traction, sucking or congestion in combination with anoxia (see also 'Asphyxia').

- *purpura* are large petechiae. They are usually larger lesions with a diameter greater than 0.5 cm.

⚠ Remember that infections and haematological disorders can cause petechiae and purpura. They may also be confused with naevi.

If the bruise is seen soon after the injury, then the site will correspond with the point of impact and will resemble the size and shape of any object causing the injury. Later, the area of bruising will be more extensive and may diffuse to a wider area. For example, a bruise to the central forehead may track down to give bilateral periorbital haematomata.

⚠ Remember that bruising in the deep tissues may not be apparent on initial examination.

The estimation of the age of a bruise is a difficult subject. Studies have disagreed on the ability to time a bruise, so it is recommended that you do not commit yourself to trying to establish the age of the bruise.

Lacerations and incised wounds
A *laceration* is a splitting of the whole skin due to blunt force but colloquially this term is used for both blunt and sharp mechanisms of injury. An *incised wound* is one in which a sharp instrument was used to injure the skin. People who do not have forensic expertise may be better to use the non-specific term 'wound' for both.

Asphyxia
Asphyxia occurs when the body is deprived of oxygen to a level at which it cannot function normally. In traumatic asphyxia, in which the chest or throat is compressed, there is increased pressure in the superior vena cava and/or neck veins. This is transmitted to the capillaries in the upper chest, neck and/or head. These petechiae are seen in the subconjunctival tissues and in the skin, particularly around the face and inside the mouth. Remember that petechiae can also have other causes, such as forceful coughing or vomiting.

Preservation of evidence

If a serious crime has been committed, the collection of evidence is the responsibility of police officers and forensic medical examiners, but health care professionals also have a duty of care to their patients to preserve evidence. In some life-threatening situations, this may not be practical, but it can be achieved in most minor injuries.

Locard's principle

The Locard's principle is that persons in contact with each other or a place will leave traces behind and will take with them traces of the person or place. These traces may be debris, hairs, fibres, body fluids, paint from vehicles, etc. Therefore, in order to preserve these traces and not contaminate them when handling the clothes of a victim or an alleged offender, the doctor or nurse should wear disposable gloves, changing them for each article touched. Each piece of clothing removed should be put into a separate *paper* bag and labelled with the following details:

- name of patient;
- date of birth of patient;
- date and time removed;
- left or right (if appropriate);
- signature of person labelling;
- signature of person to whom the specimen bag is handed (usually a police officer).

All gloves used should also be bagged and labelled. The same principles apply if a foreign body is removed from a wound.

LEGAL REPORTS

A sample legal report is shown in Figure 16.1.

These may be requested for:

- police statements;
- criminal proceedings;
- third-party claims;
- complaints;
- litigation.

STOP Whenever you are asked for a report, ask for senior advice.

The basic style is the same. Always have the report typed and keep a copy. Avoid technical medical terms or explain them in brackets (e.g. use 'hand bone' instead of 'metacarpal'). If you use professional terminology, you will be more likely to be called to court to explain it to the jury. For police statements, the description of the medical treatment does not have to be detailed, e.g. 'drips were inserted, a dressing applied and the plastic surgeon was called'.

Appropriate *consent* for disclosure of information should usually be obtained (see above).

PRIVATE AND CONFIDENTIAL REPORT

NAME OF CHILD: **DOB:**

ADDRESS:

DATE OF ATTENDANCE: **TIME OF ATTENDANCE:**

(Main part of report)

This report was **prepared at the request of** . . . .

for use in . . . .

I was **on duty as** a Senior House Officer/Registrar/Staff Nurse/GP **in** the Accident and

Emergency Department/Minor Injury Unit of the . . . . **Hospital/Clinic**

when (name) **attended.** He/she was **accompanied by** (relationship) (name). **At** . . . .

hours I assessed . . . . The **history** given to me by . . . . was

. . . .

I asked (specific question) and the reply was . . . . On examination I found

. . . . (include important negatives)

I **ordered X-Rays** of . . . .

My **conclusion** was (diagnosis or differential diagnosis).

Summarize **management and disposal** including any advice and/or appointment given.

(Space for signature)

Name in full followed by qualifications

Professional address

Date report signed

Figure 16.1 A sample legal report.

ATTENDANCE AT COURT

Attendance at court will rarely be required for minor trauma, especially if your statement or report is simple, using terminology that does not need explanation to a lay person. Most reports from doctors are accepted as fact and agreed by both sides, so the appearance of the doctor as a witness is not necessary.

If you are summonsed as a witness, ask for case-specific guidance from someone with court experience (your consultant). The general principles to be followed are:

- read your notes and report the day before the court appearance;
- dress in a professional manner;
- arrive at court at least 15 minutes before the required time and report to the clerk of the court;
- when giving evidence, speak loudly and clearly, addressing all remarks to the magistrate or judge;
- address magistrates as 'Sir' or 'Madam', and judges as 'Your Honour';
- only give the facts of your examination – you are not an expert witness and should avoid being led into giving opinions (say 'That is a question that you would need to address to an expert witness', if pushed).

Practical procedures

INTRODUCTION

Many children object to practical procedures, even if not painful. This, therefore, generates a lot of anxiety in parents and staff alike. Look confident at all times, since apprehension appears to be partly contagious!

It is important to prepare for and perform procedures swiftly. In particular, do not explain the procedure to the child, then leave them worrying about it while you go and do something else. Occasionally, sedation may be required but psychological techniques often will enable you to accomplish the task (*see Chapter 3 'Pain Management' for tips*).

EXAMINATION OF THE EARS, NOSE AND THROAT

Many children dislike examination of their ears, nose and throat (ENT). This is often best left until last. The following clinches are designed to prevent the strongest of children escaping! This is important, to both prevent the child being hurt by being poked by your equipment, and to make the examination as rapid as possible. The skills of a strong nurse can be invaluable!

Ears

Sit the child sideways on the adult's lap, asking them to 'cuddle' the child with one of their hands holding the child's arm, and their other hand over the child's head, as shown in Figure 17.1. The child faces the opposite way for examination of the other side.

Nose and throat

Sit the child on the adult's lap, facing you. The adult is asked to put one of their arms across both of the child's, and the other hand across its forehead, as shown in Figure 17.2.

In order to obtain a view of the throat, try to get the tongue depressor between the teeth. If the jaw shuts, persistent firm pressure will result in the child eventually giving way. You can then advance the tongue depressor on to the tongue.

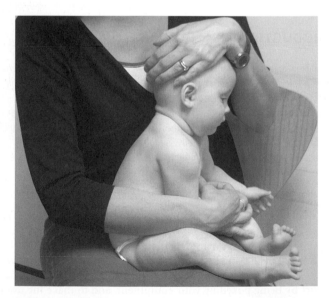

Figure 17.1 Ear examination.

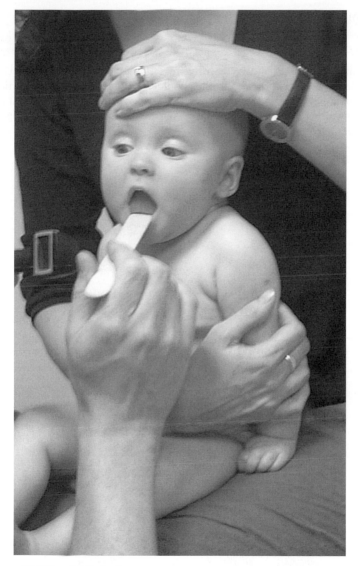

Figure 17.2 Throat examination.

SLINGS

Broad arm sling

Using a triangular bandage, place it across the chest as shown in Figure 17.3. Take the bottom corner up to the shoulder on the affected side, and tie a knot at the side of the neck with the remaining corner (Figure 17.4). At the elbow, bring the free flap across and pin to the front of the sling (Figure 17.5).

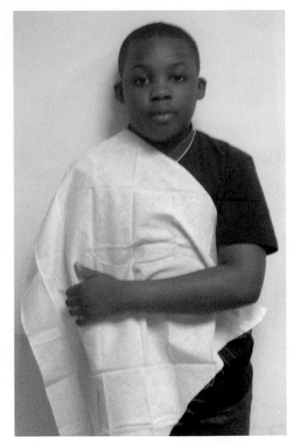

Figure 17.3 Application of a broad arm sling (step 1).

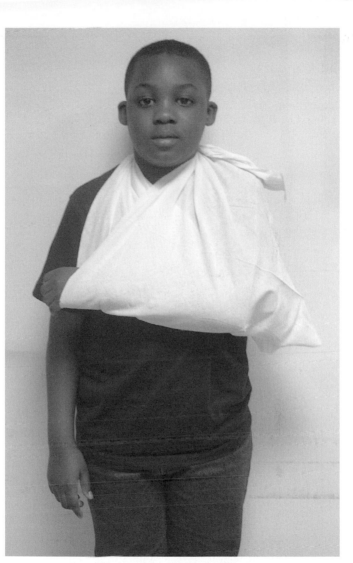

Figure 17.4 Application of a broad arm sling (step 2).

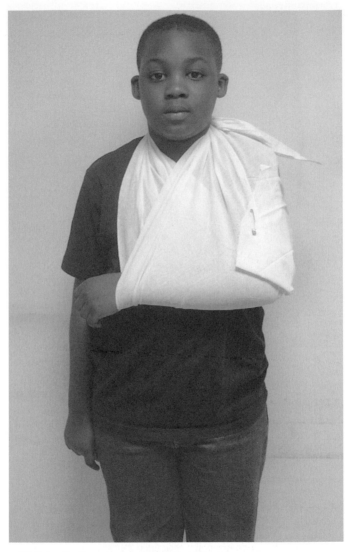

Figure 17.5 Application of a broad arm sling (step 3).

High arm sling

Using a triangular bandage, place it across the chest, over the injured arm, as shown in Figure 17.6. Take the bottom corner under the arm, up to the shoulder on the affected side and tie a knot to the side of the neck (Figure 17.7). Tie and secure as for the broad arm sling.

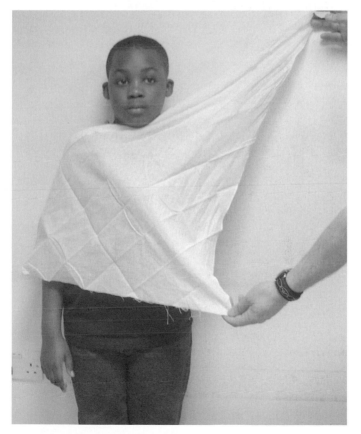

Figure 17.6 Application of a high arm sling (step 1).

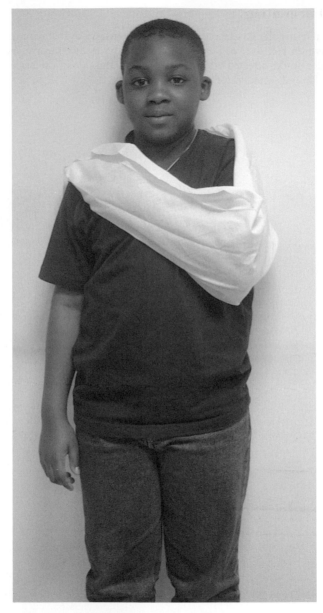

Figure 17.7 Application of a high arm sling (step 2).

'Collar and cuff'

Place a foam (e.g. Collar and Cuff™) or a long bandage around the neck, keeping one side long and the hand partially elevated. Wrap the short end around the wrist on the affected side. Bring the long end across, meeting above the wrist, and tie around all three layers (Figure 17.8). Then cut off any excess foam or bandage.

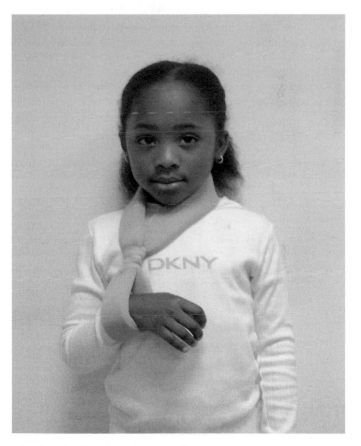

Figure 17.8 Application of a collar and cuff.

NEIGHBOUR STRAPPING

Place some folded gauze between the affected finger and a neighbouring finger, for padding. Then place tapes across the proximal and middle phalanges, avoiding the proximal and distal interphalangeal joints, to permit movement of the joints, as shown in Figure 17.9.

'BLANKET WRAP' FOR IMMOBILIZATION FOR PROCEDURES ON THE HEAD OR FACE

Unfortunately, it is sometimes necessary to wrap the child up to perform a very short procedure quickly. Most parents understand that, for a quick procedure, it is better to achieve what you want to do safely, and in the shortest time possible.

⚠ If the procedure is going to take longer than a minute or so, consider conscious sedation (see Chapter 3).

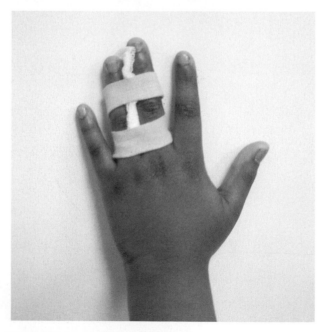

Figure 17.9 Application of neighbour strapping.

First lay the child on a blanket. Then wrap one side of the blanket diagonally across the child, incorporating the body and one arm, as shown in, then wrap the other side around to include the other arm, leaving only the head out (Figure 17.10).

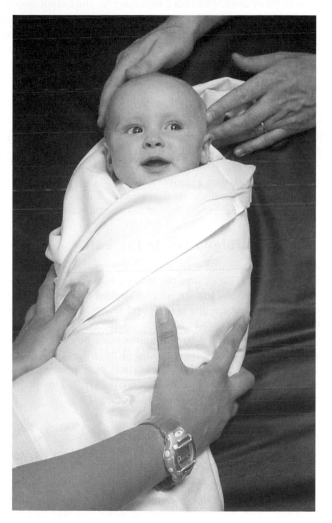

Figure 17.10 A blanket wrap for very short procedures.

FOREIGN BODIES

Removal of nasal foreign body

'The kissing technique' is a humane little technique, which unfortunately is not well known, but obviates the need for instrumentation or general anaesthesia in many cases. The added bonus is that the parent does it all!

Tell the child that 'mummy/daddy is going to give him a big kiss'. Step 1: ask the parent to sit the child on their lap sideways on, with the affected nostril against their chest. It is worth having a tissue handy to catch the offending article! Step 2: the parent occludes the unaffected nostril with a finger. Step 3: they seal their mouth over the child's and deliver a short, sharp puff. If a parent is unable to understand this, a bag and mask device can deliver the same effect.

The force of the air going up through the nasopharynx forces the foreign body down the nostril. Sometimes more than one puff is necessary actually to eject it out of the nares. The child usually does not mind, if you make a game out of it.

If this technique fails, then a blanket wrap (as above) may be necessary to remove the foreign body with some fine forceps. If it is difficult to retrieve, refer to ENT because it hurts the child, and risks further damage or aspiration.

Removal of a foreign body in the ear

There are many techniques for removing a foreign body in the ear. Small right-angled forceps (Tilley's forceps) may be used for pieces of paper or cotton wool. Alternatively, suction may be applied by using a fine suction catheter. Also, irrigation using a syringe and warm water may be used for small objects (e.g. insects).

The following technique is useful for rounded objects, such as beads. Straighten out a paper clip, leaving a bend in the middle. Make an angled 'hoop' at one end by bending it back on itself, taking care to ensure the sharp end does not protrude, as shown in Figure 17.11. This shape is ideal for manoeuvring behind the object, then scooping it out.

Removal of a foreign body in the eye

See also Chapter 5 'Head and Facial Injuries', for further management.

If a foreign body is located, most younger children will need to be referred to an ophthalmologist. For older children, instil topical anaesthetic drops, and then remove it using a moistened cotton wool bud. If this fails, in a cooperative child, use the 'scoop' of the bevel of a standard needle, by scraping gently, parallel to the corneal surface.

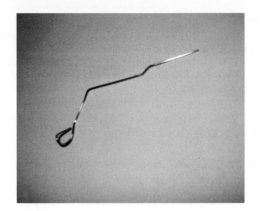

Figure 17.11 A paper clip bent into a scoop for removal of foreign bodies in the ear.

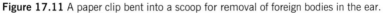

IRRIGATION OF THE EYES

See also Chapter 5 'Head and Facial Injuries', for further management.

Unlike commercially available 'eye baths', copious water is actually required to relieve symptoms from chemicals or dust. This requires a litre or more of normal saline IV solution, run through a giving set, and run as a steady stream over the affected eye(s).

REDUCTION OF A 'PULLED ELBOW'

This common injury is sustained when a toddler is pulled by the hand (see Chapter 8 'Injuries of the Upper Limb').

⚠ **Make sure the mechanism of injury is classical, and the child is the right age group, before attempting reduction.**

Given the above precaution, reduction may be attempted without an X-ray. You must explain what you are about to do to the parent, in the most reassuring terms! It is important to warn them that the child will cry.

Step 1: sit the child on the parent's lap, sideways on. Step 2: put one thumb over the head of the radius and with your other hand, hold the child's hand. Step 3: Fully supinate and pronate the forearm. You may feel a click, either beneath your thumb, or transmitted down to the hand. Step 4:

If not, try to bring the arm into full extension and supination (there may be resistance), and then return the arm to its original position. Sometimes the click is felt at this stage. Step 5: whether or not a click was felt, leave the room at this stage to allow the child to settle down and play with some toys, to see if they start using the arm. Review the child after 10 minutes. See Chapter 8 for further management.

TREPHINING A NAIL

Crush injuries to fingertips are common, and may cause a subungual haematoma (see Chapter 9 'Hand Injuries'). Trephining the nail releases the blood and is a very satisfying procedure because of the instant relief of symptoms.

To do this, the nail is literally melted by a hot metal wire, to make a hole through which the blood drains (beware, it often spurts out like a fountain!). If performed quickly and efficiently, there is only a second or so of pain. It is, therefore, imperative that a second, strong member of staff holds the child's hand down to prevent sudden withdrawal.

Your place of work may have a purpose-made battery-operated device in which a fine wire heats up, but if not, a paper clip can be used. A green needle will do the job, but is at increased risk of penetrating the nailbed and causing further pain or harm. When the metal is red hot, puncture the nail with one firm, swift action, withdrawing quickly. Do not be put off by burning and hissing!

The paper clip technique involves straightening out one side of a paper clip and applying some Elastoplast to the remaining clip to prevent you burning your fingers as it heats up. Heat the straight part in a flame (paraffin oil lamp or cigarette lighter), then proceed as above.

WOUND MANAGEMENT

Wound irrigation

See Chapter 4 'Wounds and Soft Tissue Injuries' for further advice about wound management.

To clean a wound adequately, irrigation with copious quantities of water is the most important principle, to decrease the bacterial load. Infiltrate the wound with local anaesthetic, if necessary. Place the affected part on a good thickness of absorbent towels. Use a 20 ml or 50 ml syringe, and a large bowl of water or saline to repeatedly flush inside the wound, or use a litre of IV saline directing the flow through a standard intravenous giving set.

Adhesive strips and glue

Adhesive strips such as Steristrips™ and tissue glue provide equal, if not better, cosmetic outcomes than sutures for many wounds. It all depends on the tension across the wound, which is only partly related to its depth, but significantly related to wound length and shape, and the direction of the wound to Langer's lines (see Chapter 4 'Wounds and Soft Tissue Injuries').

Both adhesive strips and glue are probably of similar efficacy, and both may be used together if a wound needs good support. Adhesive strips cannot be used on hairy areas. Tissue glue cannot be used near the eyes.

Applying adhesive strips

These should be laid perpendicular to the wound, bringing a small amount of tension to the wound edges to ensure adequate opposition but not bunching up of the edges. For children it is worth laying extra strips at 90°, over either end of the main strips. Tincture of benzoin can help stick them down, especially if the skin is sweaty or the wound moist. N.B. Be careful not to get it in the wound as it stings.

Circumferential strips should not be applied around fingertips. Apply them longitudinally to allow for swelling.

Applying tissue glue

Tissue glue is not totally painless – there is burning during the exothermic reaction as it hardens. However, it is a concept that seems to appeal to children, thus overcoming their apprehension. N.B. Sterile gloves stick easily to glue!

Take care only to place the glue as a seal over the top of the wound. If it drips between the wound edges, it will have the opposite effect of preventing healing.

⚠ **Care must be taken to avoid the eyes.**

If any glue is dropped near the eyes, stop and wipe *immediately* with a wet swab. If this does not work, it will gradually come off over the coming days, but further attempts at removal before this time are likely to result in more damage.

Local infiltration of anaesthesia

If there is no regional block for a particular area (see below), anaesthetic agents may be infiltrated locally. The choice of anaesthetic is explained in Table 17.1.

 If the toxic dose of local anaesthetic is likely to be exceeded, the child will need general anaesthesia for wound repair.

Table 17.1 Choice of local anaesthetic agents

Drug	Toxic dose	Indications
1% lignocaine	3 mg/kg (= 0.3 mls/kg)	Local wound infiltration. Onset 2–3 mins. Offset variable but usually < 1 hour
2% lignocaine	3 mg/kg (= 0.15 ml/kg)	More effective than 1% if able to stay within toxic dose
Lignocaine 1% with adrenaline (1:200,000)	6 mg/kg of lignocaine component (= 0.6 mls/kg)	Vascular areas e.g. face, scalp. DO NOT use in end-organs, e.g. fingers, penis, pinna
Bupivacaine	2 mg/kg (= 0.4 mls/kg of 0.5% solution)	Longer acting than lignocaine. Onset 5 mins. Offset 1–4 hours

Infiltration of local anaesthesia is generally very safe, but overdose may result in facial tingling, cardiac arrhythmias and seizures.

(STOP) **Will the child cooperate or will they need sedation or general anaesthesia? (See Chapter 3 'Pain Management'.)**

For a wound, after thorough cleaning, inject anaesthetic along the wound edges using a blue (23 gauge), or orange (25 gauge) needle, passing the needle straight into the subcutaneous tissues through the wound rather than through the intact skin, which is more painful. Slow injection will decrease stinging.

Always inject further anaesthetic through the area you have just anaesthetized, waiting half a minute if there are few injections and the child is cooperative.

Suturing

For a full description of the indications for, and pitfalls regarding, suturing, see Chapter 4 'Wounds and Soft Tissue Injuries'.

The technique for inserting interrupted sutures is described below. When choosing suture material, bear in mind that absorbable sutures are useful for avoiding suture removal in children. Non-absorbable sutures should be used in the face, however, to avoid suture marks.

⚠ **Think twice before suturing a wound on the face – are you sufficiently skilled? (See Chapter 5 'Head and Facial Injuries'.)**

The size of suture depends on the amount of tension or wear and tear over the area, but should be the smallest size possible, e.g. 3-0 or 4-0 for scalps, 4-0 or 5-0 for limbs, and 5-0 or 6-0 for faces.

Step 1: Pick up the needle with the suture holder, as shown in Figure 17.12. The needle holder should be placed about two-thirds of the way back along the needle.

Step 2: Introduce the needle to the skin at 90° and aim vertically down to include sufficient tissue to provide support for the suture, and avoid tension on the wound, as shown in Figure 17.13. Hold the tissue with forceps, avoiding crushing the edge of the wound. Push the needle through, following the curve of the needle. Pull most of the thread through, allowing a small length to remain for tying. Pick up this end with your needle holder in your right hand.

Step 3: Tie a triple knot to secure the suture. Now pick up the long needle end of the thread in your left hand and wrap it twice around the needle

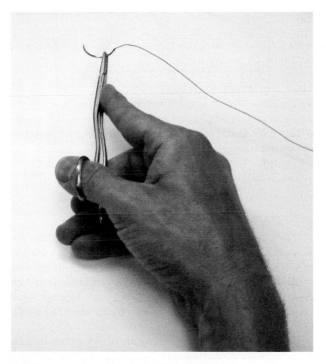

Figure 17.12 The correct position for holding a needle.

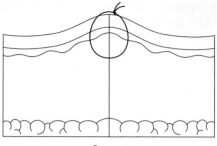

Correct

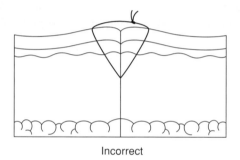

Incorrect

Figure 17.13 A cross-section of skin tissues demonstrating the correct (and incorrect) placement of a suture.

holder clockwise, as shown in Figure 17.14. Without letting go, let the thread slide off the needle holder and pull it tight to form a knot, as shown in Figure 17.15. Do not leave the knot over the middle of the wound, but bring it to the side. Ensure that the wound edges are not inverted, everted or under tension. This leads to scarring.

Step 4: Repeat, wrapping anticlockwise once around the needle holder and tie.

Step 5: The same but wrap clockwise again. Cut the ends long enough to permit grasping when removing, particularly for scalp sutures in children with dark hair.

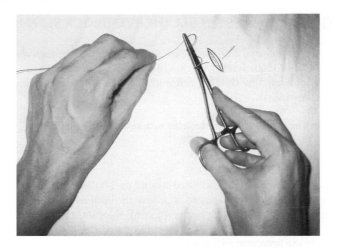

Figure 17.14 Wrapping the suture thread around the needle holder.

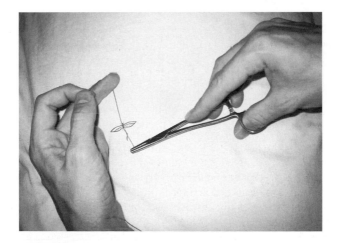

Figure 17.15 Tying a knot.

REGIONAL ANAESTHESIA (NERVE BLOCKS)

Techniques of regional anaesthesia are usually easy to learn and, once mastered, can be very satisfying. Injection of anaesthetic away from the affected site is well tolerated by children and multiple injections or conscious sedation can be avoided.

⚠ **Check for sensory deficit associated with injury *before* injecting.**

Digital block

The four digital nerves are distributed around the phalanx as shown in Figure 17.16. Inject 1 ml of 2% lignocaine as close to the bone as possible, along two perpendicular sides, aspirating before injecting. Repeat on the other side.

⚠ **Never use lignocaine with adrenaline to inject a digit!**

After performing the block, consider the use of a tourniquet to decrease bleeding and prolong the duration of anaesthesia.

⚠ **A tourniquet should not be used for more than 20 minutes.**

Make a glove tourniquet by placing the hand in a small disposable glove after cutting the glove fingertip. Roll back the glove fingertip to the base.

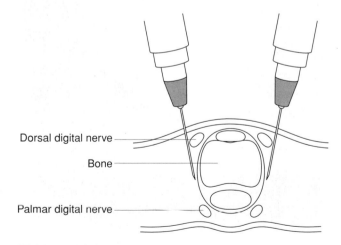

Dorsal digital nerve

Bone

Palmar digital nerve

Figure 17.16 The digital block technique.

Auricular nerve block

This block is invaluable for procedures on the lower half of the pinna, in particular for removing embedded earrings.

The earlobe is often swollen and may be infected and extremely tender; injecting anaesthetic into the earlobe is very painful and difficult. However, injecting away from the ear is usually well tolerated. The block works up to around halfway up the pinna. It blocks branches of the greater auricular and auriculotemporal nerves.

Using about 2 ml of 2% lignocaine, the needle enters the skin 1 cm below where the earlobe joins the face (near the angle of the jaw, as shown in Figure 17.17). Direct half the volume anteriorly towards the tragus, and half posteriorly, back towards the mastoid.

Femoral nerve and 'three in one' nerve blocks

Either of these blocks is used to provide analgesia for a fractured shaft of femur. The block should be performed before X-ray, or application of traction (see Chapter 10 'Injuries of the Lower Limb').

A femoral nerve block uses a syringe and needle directed vertically downwards. A 'three in one' block, via an intravenous cannula instead of a needle, is a less painful technique, and avoids inadvertently hitting the nerve with a needle.

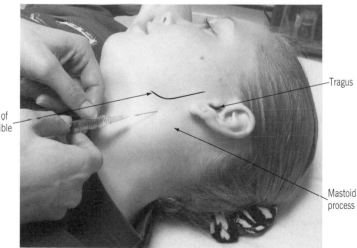

Figure 17.17 The inferior auricular block technique.

⚠ These blocks take about 20 minutes to work, so IV morphine or intranasal diamorphine may be required in the interim (see Chapter 3 'Pain Management').

The femoral nerve block

Use 0.5% bupivacaine with a volume of around 2 mg/kg (i.e. 0.4 ml/kg). Draw up the anaesthetic in a syringe then attach a 21 Ch needle. Partially abduct the leg and locate the femoral pulse and the inguinal ligament. For a child under 8 years old, enter the skin 1 cm lateral to the pulse, just below the inguinal ligament, and for children over 8 years, enter 2 cm lateral to the pulse.

Aim directly downwards as far as you would for arterial or venous sampling, aspirating regularly. If there is no flushback, slowly inject the anaesthetic.

Modified femoral nerve block ('three in one' block)

This technique blocks the femoral, obturator and lateral cutaneous nerves. Use the same volume of anaesthetic and landmarks as for the femoral block, but use a 20 Ch cannula. Direct the cannula towards the mid-clavicular line at 45° to the skin, as shown in Figure 17.18. Once it is halfway in, try to

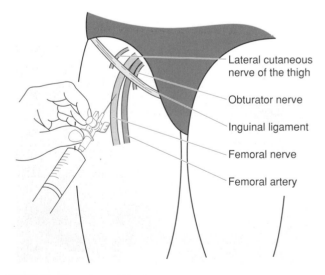

Lateral cutaneous nerve of the thigh

Obturator nerve

Inguinal ligament

Femoral nerve

Femoral artery

Figure 17.18 The 'three in one' block technique.

advance the cannula over the needle. If you are in the right place (a potential space overlying the psoas fascia), it should advance freely. Check there is no flushback, then attach your syringe and inject the anaesthetic. This should inject freely, as if into a vein.

Foot blocks

The nerve distribution to the foot is individually quite variable, but the use of a block is much easier than local infiltration into the sole of the foot.

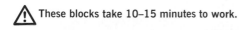 These blocks take 10–15 minutes to work.

Dorsum of the foot
Infiltrate 1 ml 2% lignocaine either side of the dorsalis pedis artery, as shown in Figure 17.19. This anaesthetizes the medial plantar nerve. Aim to puncture the skin only once, with repositioning of the needle by withdrawing slightly.

Medial border of the sole
Infiltrate 1 ml 2% lignocaine either side of the posterior tibial artery, behind the medial malleolus, as shown in Figure 17.20, using the same technique as above. This anaesthetizes the posterior tibial nerve.

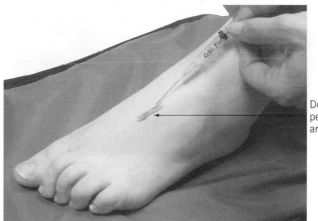

Dorsalis pedis artery

Figure 17.19 The technique for blocking the dorsum of the foot.

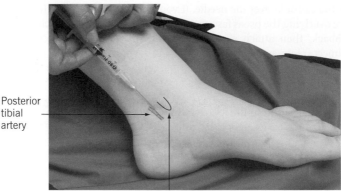

Posterior
tibial
artery

Medial malleolus

Figure 17.20 The technique for blocking the medial border of the sole.

Lateral border of the sole

Infiltrate 3–5 ml of 1% lignocaine between the lateral malleolus and the Achilles tendon, in a line, a few centimetres higher than the tip of the lateral malleolus (Figure 17.21). This anaesthetizes the sural nerve.

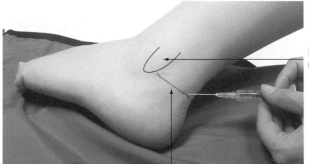

Lateral
malleolus

Area of infiltration from lateral
malleolus back to Achilles tendon

Figure 17.21 The technique for blocking the lateral border of the sole.

Index